**DO NOT REMOVE
CARDS FROM POCKET**

Nutrition
FOR THE
Prime
OF
Your Life

Books by Annette B. Natow and Jo-Ann Heslin

No Nonsense Nutrition for Your Baby's First Year
Geriatric Nutrition

Nutrition
FOR THE
Prime
OF
Your Life

Annette B. Natow, Ph.D., R.D.

Jo-Ann Heslin, M.A., R.D.

McGraw-Hill Book Company

New York · St. Louis · San Francisco · Bogotá
Guatemala · Hamburg · Lisbon · Madrid
Mexico · Montreal · Panama · Paris · San Juan
São Paulo · Tokyo · Toronto

"Better Butter" from *Laurel's Kitchen: A Handbook for Vegetarian Cookery & Nutrition* by Laurel Robertson, Carol Flinders, and Bronwen Godfrey © 1976 by Nilgiri Press, Petaluma, California 94953. Reprinted with permission.

"Nutritional Analysis of Fast Foods" from Young, E. A., "Perspective on Fast Foods," *Dietetic Currents,* Ross Laboratories, Columbus, Ohio, 1981. Reprinted with permission.

1 2 3 4 5 6 7 8 9 D O C D O C 8 7 6 5 4 3

ISBN 0-07-028414-8

LIBRARY OF CONGRESS CATALOGING IN PUBLICATION DATA
Natow, Annette B.
    Nutrition for the prime of your life.

    1. Middle age—Nutrition.   I. Heslin, Jo-Ann.
II. Title.
TX361.M47N37   1983   613.2   82-17130
ISBN 0-07-028414-8

Book design by Roberta Rezk.

To
      Harry, Joe, Edna, and Irwin
              A.B.N.

Joseph, who nourishes my growth
               J.H.

ACKNOWLEDGMENTS

We would like to thank the following people for all their assistance: Ralph Kamhi; Marilyn Kirshenbaum; Enid Lederer; Martin Lefkowitz, M.D.; Allen Natow, M.D.; Laura N. Lefkowitz for typing the manuscript; and our families Harry, Steven, Laura, Allen, Joseph, Marty, Kristen and Karen for their support and encouragement.

While many things contribute to health—sleep, fresh air, and exercise, for instance—the foremost consideration is food.

Mary Swartz Rose,
Feeding the Family, 1919

Contents

Introduction

When Annette Natow was growing up, her mother often told her stories about her own childhood and the wonderful Irish housekeeper, Maggie, who had lived with them and helped raise the large family of eight children. It seems that Maggie was wise, witty, and could also predict events as disparate as the weather tomorrow or which child would be likely to lose his or her scarf that afternoon. The children were amazed by her powers and when they asked her how she could predict so many things accurately, Maggie would answer in a soft brogue, "Wait until you are forty years old. . . ."

Maggie was right, with age and experience come wisdom and an understanding of how to deal with the realities of life. You who are forty, forty-five, fifty, or more have learned to value your health and well-being. You know that it is vital to take care of your body so that you can enjoy a rich, productive life for many more years. You know that adequate exercise and rest, mental stimulation, and medical care are all essential to your well-being. You also have heard many times that you are what you eat. In other words, the food and drink you enjoy in your meals and snacks becomes part of every cell of your body and also provides you with energy you need for living. Nourishing your body is vital but at the same time frought with misunderstanding: You hear and read about the latest nutrient or food—be it fiber, zinc, vitamin E, or ginseng root—and all the wonderful things it can do for you. You are also cautioned to reduce your intake of sugar, salt, and fat.

You may be advised to reduce the amount of some kinds of fat you eat while at the same time increasing the amount of other types of fat. It's hard to know what to do.

To compound this confusing information you are beginning to notice changes in your body: your hair may be graying, there may be more "laugh lines" around your eyes, your waistline may be spreading. These are outward signs that your body is changing. Change is a part of life; in fact nothing is as constant as change.

You'll be reassured to learn that although change is a natural part of life and that some change is inevitable as you get older, your lifestyle, particularly food and exercise habits, can help to minimize some of the less desirable changes and enable you to enjoy a healthy, active, well-functioning body throughout your life. Remember, the best is still to come, but don't sit back, *get up and enjoy it!*

We wrote this book to help you do just that. We will present all the facts as we know them (and we are trained, experienced nutritionists, one of us close to forty, one close to fifty) about the various nutrients you need for optimum health and show you that there are many paths you can take to reach good nutrition. We will show you how to choose the proper foods and plan meals to insure that you are getting all the essential nutrients. This is possible for most of you who are healthy and want to stay that way and for those of you who have some medical problem that can be helped by good nutrition. We'll also give you a few of our easy, often used, favorite recipes so that your food will taste great.

Our book is written in question-and-answer form. Most of these questions are ones we have been asked again and again in the course of our work and social life (you can imagine how popular we are at parties and other functions when the guests find out that we are nutritionists). Each question is answered as completely as possible in easy-to-understand language (you won't have to reach for a medical dictionary) and we'll give you useful and practical suggestions. We did this so that if you have a particular problem, for example indigestion, you can look that subject up in the index and find out what you want to know. The index will prove very helpful since we have discussed the same topic in many places throughout the book.

Of course we hope that you will read through most of the chapters. Then you too will have lots to tell your family and friends about nutrients, calories, losing weight, vegetarianism, drug and food interactions, food and exercise, and much more. Look through the table of contents to see what we mean.

We feel that not only is food the most important environmental factor in health, it is one thing you can do something about right now. We know that you will find this book a practical, usable guide. We have tried to cover a broad range of subjects and hope we have provided the answers to your questions. If there is an area or a specific question we have overlooked, please let us know. We learn a lot from our readers and friends.

Nutrition
FOR THE
Prime
OF
Your Life

1

The Lowdown on Nutrients

Many magazine and newspaper articles offer you suggestions about what to eat—high protein, low protein, high carbohydrate, low carbohydrate, high fiber, and sometimes a combination of these. It's hard to know what's best. You may think that you can just continue to eat the way you always have—it's all food, isn't it? Well, it's not that simple. There's a lot to know about what's right to eat, and starting here you can learn.

The kinds of foods we eat are alike in some ways: they give us energy (calories is another word for energy) and they satisfy our hunger. But in other important ways, foods are different from each other because each food is a unique mixture of nutrients—protein, carbohydrate, fat, vitamins, and minerals. Meat is a mixture of protein, fat, vitamins, and minerals, while fruits are basically carbohydrates, vitamins, minerals, plus fiber and water. These last two, while not nutrients in the strict sense, are essential for health.

Did you ever really think about what you eat each day? On the following page there is a little quiz to help you become more aware of the way you eat.

1

FOOD INTAKE QUIZ

Circle the appropriate answer to each question.

1. I eat two or more servings of vegetables every day. (Example: ½ cup broccoli, ½ cup carrots, ½ cup zucchini, 1 tomato) Yes No Sometimes

2. I eat two or more servings of fruit each day. (Example: banana, mango, apple, grapes) Yes No Sometimes

3. I eat one serving of vitamin-C-rich food each day. (Example: orange, grapefruit, tomato, or their juices, strawberries, cantaloupe, or coleslaw) Yes No Sometimes

4. I drink two glasses of milk each day, or I eat two servings of dairy foods each day. (Example: cheese, yogurt, custard) Yes No Sometimes

5. I eat at least two servings of lean meat, fish, poultry, dried peas or beans, or nuts. Yes No Sometimes

6. I eat no more than three to four eggs each week. Yes No Sometimes

7. I eat four or more servings of bread, cereals, rice, noodles, or pasta each day. Yes No Sometimes

8. I eat whole-grain breads and cereals. Yes No Sometimes

9. I eat no more than one serving of cake, cookies, pastries, similar baked goods, or candy each day. Yes No Sometimes

10. I limit my use of salt and salty foods each day. (Example: ham, bacon, snack chips, pickles, canned or dry soup) Yes No Sometimes

11. I limit my use of fats and oils each day. (Example: butter, margarine, salad dressing, and fried foods) Yes No Sometimes

12. I drink no more than two   Yes   No   Sometimes
    alcoholic drinks each day.
    (Example: beer, wine, cocktail)

For every question answered *yes*, give yourself 2 points.
For every question answered *sometimes* you get 1 point.
You get no points for those questions answered *no*.

Now rate your diet!

Points
   24 to 18—Keep it up; you're eating well!
   17 to 12—Not too bad, but there's definitely room for
           improvement.
   11 to 5—Watch it, your diet needs work.
   5 or less—Danger! Resolve to change your ways today!

✳ What is a nutrient?

Protein, fat, carbohydrate, vitamins, and minerals are nutrients. You eat these substances in food. They supply you
with energy, provide for growth, repair your body, and also
regulate body processes. Water and fiber, while not really
nutrients, are used by the body in some similar ways.

Steak is a mixture of protein, fat, vitamins, and minerals.
Eating it not only gives you energy but also raw materials for
building body tissues and vitamins and minerals. (Let's not
forget that eating steak is fun; it tastes good.) Other foods you
enjoy contain carbohydrates—sugars and starches. These
carbohydrates along with protein and fat contain energy, the
chart "Energy Nutrients" summarizes important information
about them. You will notice that vitamins and minerals are
not on the chart because they do not contain energy. You
need vitamins and minerals to help your body use the energy
in carbohydrate, fat, and protein but vitamins and minerals
themselves do not yield energy. (Remember this the next
time a friend tells you that he gained weight from taking a
vitamin supplement.) You'll read more about these essential
regulators in Chapter 2.

ENERGY NUTRIENTS

Nutrient	Sources	Functions
Protein	Meat, fish, poultry, milk, eggs, dried peas and beans, tofu, peanuts and other nuts	Building blocks for growth and repair of body; makes enzymes, antibodies, hormones
Fat	Butter, margarine, whole milk, eggs, meat, cheese	Cushions and protects organs; helps regulate body temperature; provides essential fatty acids
Carbohydrate	Sugar, honey, bread, noodles, rice, pasta, dried peas and beans	Forms body substances; maintains normal body metabolism

PROTEIN

* Is protein the most important nutrient?

Protein, or more precisely, the *amino acids* that make up protein are important nutrients. Protein is found in every cell of the body and all of the body substances too. Urine and bile are the two exceptions, they don't normally contain protein.

Many people believe that protein is the key to good health and that a large protein intake is important for a slim, vigorous, youthful body. The key word in the preceding sentence is "large," because while some protein is essential, it is neither necessary nor desirable to eat large amounts. In fact, most of us eat two to three times as much as we need. The extra protein, the amount left over after the essential uses (outlined in table "Energy Nutrients") are taken care of, is simply used for energy or stored as body fat. As an energy source, protein is not as efficient as fat or carbohydrate.

* How much protein should I eat?

The answer to this really depends on what kinds of protein foods you eat. If you usually eat protein from animal sources—meat, fish, poultry, eggs, milk, cheese—you are eating proteins of high biological value. This means that these proteins are similar in composition to the protein in your body so that you can easily convert them to body tissue. If all the protein you ate came from animal sources you would need only about 25 grams a day (the amount in five teaspoons of pure protein). This is just enough to make up for the protein lost from the body each day.

Practically speaking, it is unwise to limit protein to such a low level because you get protein from many different foods, not only animal foods. Some of this protein is from vegetables, the composition of which is not as similar to your body. Think about a carrot and a cow. Which of these does your body more closely resemble?

There are times when you need additional protein. Infections, injury, psychological stress, even confinement to bed increases the amount of protein you need. So, to be on the safe side, it's a good idea to eat about 50 or 60 grams of protein daily from a variety of sources. The chart "Protein in Foods" will show you how much protein you get from different foods. You will see that if you drink some milk (one or two cups), eat some meat, fish, poultry, or beans (two 3- or 4-ounce servings) and perhaps an egg or some nuts along with bread and vegetables, you will easily eat more than enough protein.

PROTEIN IN FOODS

Food	Portion	Grams of protein
Apple	1	Trace
Bread, white	1 slice	2
Green beans	1 cup	2
Beans sprouts, mung, cooked	1 cup	3
Alfalfa sprouts, raw	1 cup	3
Bread, whole-wheat	1 slice	3
Bacon	2 slices	4
Sunflower seeds	2 tablespoons	4
Potato	1 baked	4
Rice, white	1 cup	4
Rice, brown	1 cup	5
Oatmeal, cooked	1 cup	5

PROTEIN IN FOODS

Food	Portion	Grams of protein
American cheese, processed	1 slice	6
Egg	1	6
Bean sprouts, soy, cooked	1 cup	7
Cheese, natural	1 ounce	7
Spaghetti	1 cup	7
Dried peas or beans, cooked	½ cup	8
Skim milk	1 cup	8
Peanut butter	2 tablespoons	8
Peanuts	¼ cup roasted	9
Walnuts	½ cup	9
Tofu	4 ounces	9
Milk, whole	1 cup	9
Milk, low-fat protein fortified	1 cup	10
Yogurt	1 cup	12
Tuna salad	½ cup	15
Cottage cheese, creamed	½ cup	15
Baked beans	1 cup	16
Pork chop	3 ounces	19
Hamburger	3 ounces	20
Sardines	3 ounces	20
Chicken	¼ chicken	21
Turkey, dark meat	4 ounces	26

* Is brewer's yeast a good protein supplement?

Brewer's yeast, along with wheat germ, vitamin E, lecithin, and bee pollen are wrongly believed to be ergogenic (energy enhancing). One tablespoon of brewer's yeast does provide approximately 16 calories in the form of protein (3.7 grams) and some B vitamins. However, there is little, if any, vitamin B_{12} in brewer's, baker's, or live yeast. ("Nutritional" or "food" yeast differs since it is grown on a vitamin B_{12} enriched culture so that the B_{12} content of the yeast is substantial.)

Since adults in the United States eat two to three times as much protein as they need each day, supplements are not something we normally recommend. Brewer's yeast is related to the dried bitter by-product of beer brewing and it is neither the most appetizing nor the most useful protein supplement.

If you like brewer's yeast, or feel it is particularly useful to you, a small daily supplement is probably not harmful. Be aware, though, that there was a reported case of fever of unknown origin in a sixty-eight-year-old man that was finally traced to a daily dose of brewer's yeast.

Go slowly if you intend to "sprinkle" your food with brewer's yeast. Some people develop excessive, uncomfortable, and embarrassing gas. Start with a half teaspoon and gradually work up to a maximum daily supplement of no more than one tablespoon.

CARBOHYDRATE

* I think carbohydrates are fattening. Do I really need to eat them?

Sugars and starches make up the carbohydrates we eat, and they are important parts of a good diet. Sugars are sometimes called "simple" carbohydrates and starches are called "complex." They have an undeserved reputation for being fattening when, ounce for ounce, they are equal to protein and much lower than fat in the calories they contain. While it is probably a good idea to use only small amounts of sugar in beverages, desserts, and pastries, other carbohydrates—sugars in fruit and milk and starches in bread, potatoes, beans and cereals—are useful in many ways. In addition to the functions of carbohydrate shown in the chart "Energy Nutrients," carbohydrate-rich food contains needed vitamins, minerals, and fiber essential to normal body functions.

* How much carbohydrate do I need each day?

Most of us eat about 200 to 300 grams of carbohydrate (sugar and starch) every day. That is more than the 100 grams needed for normal body metabolism. Reducing the amount of carbohydrate you eat to less than 100 grams a day, as is often suggested in weight-loss diets, is unwise and unnecessary. Besides being needed for normal body function, carbohydrate foods contain many other essential nutrients. In short, they are good for you and also low or fairly low in calories. Their reputation as being fattening is undeserved. This is due more to the way carbohydrate foods are prepared and served (with oil, sour cream, or butter) than the calorie count of the food itself. The chart "Carbohydrates in Foods" that follows will give you the calorie content of some carbohydrate foods. The chart also gives the grams of carbohydrate in these foods.

For good health, it's better to eat foods rich in starch like bread, cereals, and potatoes instead of foods high in sugar like candy, cake, syrup, and sweetened soft drinks.

Carbohydrates in Foods

Food	Portion	Grams of carbohydrate	Calories
All-Bran	1 cup	40	129
Apple	1	22	87
Bagel	1	30	165
Banana	1	33	127
Beans	½ cup	21	118
Biscuit	1	16	129
Blueberries	1 cup	21	87
Bread, cracked wheat	1 slice	12	60
Bread, white	1 slice	12	62
Bread, whole-wheat	1 slice	11	56
Cantaloupe	¼ melon	7	30
Caramels	1 ounce (3 pieces)	21	113
Cola	12 ounces	36	129
Corn	1 ear	22	94
Cornflakes	1 ounce	24	109
Corn grits	½ cup	13	61
Dates	5	36	137
Farina	½ cup	14	67

CARBOHYDRATES IN FOODS

Food	Portion	Grams of carbohydrate	Calories
Fig Newton	1 cookie	11	50
Ginger ale	12 ounces	34	136
Green beans	½ cup	21	110
Graham crackers	2	10	54
Granola	1 ounce	19	128
Grape-Nuts	1 ounce	23	100
Grapefruit	½	11	41
Hamburger roll	1	16	89
Ice cream, vanilla, soft	½ cup	34	160
Kool-Aid	1 cup	25	100
Marshmallow	1	6	25
Matzoh	1 piece	25	117
Melba toast	1 slice	3	15
Muffin, bran	1	17	104
Noodles	½ cup	18	100
Oatmeal	½ cup	13	74
Oatmeal cookie	1	12	80
Peas	½ cup	8	46
Potato, baked	1	21	95
Rice	½ cup	18	82
Saltines	2	5	28
Shredded wheat	1 biscuit	20	89
Spaghetti	½ cup	17	83
Sweet potato	1	32	141
Sweet roll	1	27	174
Tang	1 cup	34	135

✳ Is white bread nutritionally equal to whole-wheat bread?

When whole wheat is refined to make white flour the bran and the wheat germ are removed. Eight vitamins and thirteen minerals are lost in the process. Enriched white bread has four of these nutrients put back in—thiamine, riboflavin, niacin, and iron. If you compare whole-wheat and enriched white bread for these four nutrients, you'll find that they are about equal. But this is only part of the comparison. While whole-wheat bread contains 15 percent fewer calories, it is a much better source of fiber, magnesium, zinc, copper, chromium, folic acid, vitamin B$_6$, vitamin K, and vitamin E.

Some people tell us they dislike whole-wheat bread and much prefer white bread. Because the benefits of whole grains are so important, why don't you try some of the newer whole-grain breads to see if you can find one you like. You must check the label. Some companies are now making "wheat" bread. This is not the same as whole wheat. On the label you'll see that whole wheat is the second, third, or fourth ingredient, which shows it isn't the main grain used. While these "wheat" breads have more fiber than white bread, they are not equal to whole wheat. Some wheaty looking dark breads are colored with caramel or raisin juice so these too contain less fiber than whole wheat.

You might be interested to know that only 23 percent of all bread baked is white bread. This is much less than in the past. Consumers are changing.

* I have a sweet tooth. Is sugar really bad for me?

Many of us worry about the amount of sugar we eat, over 130 pounds a year. A recent survey showed that 91 percent of the people questioned agreed that everyone should eat less sugar. This was in spite of the fact that 70 percent reported eating cake, pie, or other sweet baked goods at least once a week. You can see that you are not alone in liking sweets and worrying about them.

Sugary foods usually offer little or no necessary nutrients along with their high calories— and we are at a time in life when our need for calories is less than before. We cannot indulge our sweet tooth too often if we want to be certain we are getting all the nutrients we need and still stay within our calorie budget. Sugary foods give us a pleasant taste and little more.

Besides supplying us with lots of unnecessary calories, sweets are a factor in tooth decay and gum disease, which is rampant in the United States. By age seventeen, each one of us averaged eight or nine teeth that were decayed, filled, or missing and loss of teeth in middle age is often due to gum disease.

You may have heard that eating a lot of sugar will cause diabetes. There is no truth to this. While it is important to eliminate sugar when you have diabetes, the sugar did not cause the disease. (Read more about diabetes in Chapter 9.) There may be some truth in the idea that eating a lot of sugar causes heart disease. (See Chapter 8 for further information on heart disease.)

If sweets please you, go ahead and enjoy them once in a while. At the same time that you are enjoying an occasional treat, try to reduce your habitual use of sugar. If you usually use two teaspoons of sugar in your beverages, reduce this amount first to one-and-a-half teaspoons and then, after a while, to one. You will get used to less sugar and you may even find that you learn to like some beverages "straight"— with no added sugar.

* Which is better, honey or sugar?

Sugar is sugar is sugar, whether it comes from a beehive, sugar beet, or sugarcane. We'd prefer that you attempt to cut down on your sugar consumption rather than worry about which sugar is best.

Honey is popular and the subtle taste difference among the varieties available can be interesting to explore. Nutritionally speaking, however, honey has no advantage over sugar and it is significantly more expensive.

Suggested as a quick energizer, honey is often used by joggers and runners. One tablespoon of honey yields 64 calories and one tablespoon of sugar 46. Both must be broken down to glucose before they can enter the bloodsteam and be used as energy. Therefore, the sugar from an apple, a spoonful of honey, or a sugar cube will be available as energy for use by the body in about the same amount of time.

While it is true that honey has greater sweetening power than sugar (about twice as sweet) it is not a concentrated source of nutrients. Even if you ate one cup of honey you would get only tiny amounts of the vitamins and minerals you need daily. (The one exception to this is vitamin B_{12}. One cup of honey does provide 50 percent of your daily need of this nutrient along with 1,031 calories!)

In the book *Folk Medicine: A Vermont Doctor's Guide to Good Health,* author Dr. Deforest Jarvis claims honey can cure bedwetting, sleeplessness, muscle cramps, and a runny nose. He further states that two tablespoons of honey at each meal will prevent migraines. Scientific medicine has refuted all these claims. To quote Dr. Frederick Stare, "This claptrap is strictly for those gullible birds stung by the honeybee."

* Is raw sugar better to eat than regular white sugar?

Raw sugar, coarse and granular, comes from the evaporation of sugarcane juice. It may not be sold in the United States unless its impurities—dirt, insect fragments, chaff—are removed.

Turbinado sugar is often erroneously thought to be raw sugar. Turbinado sugar is actually a refined sugar that has been processed to remove impurities and most of the natural molasses. It is tan or brown in color and ground to a coarse crystal. It is made of glucose and fructose like table sugar and differs from it only in its coarser shape, slight percent of molasses, and its much higher cost per pound.

* Is it a good idea to eat sugared cereal for breakfast?

Many presweetened ready-to-eat breakfast cereals are very high in sugar. So high, in fact, that they taste more like candy than cereal. Many presweetened cereals contain an average of two teaspoons of sugar or more in each serving. Many people enjoy these and won't eat cereal any other way.

When we try to improve the quality of our diet, one of the things we aim for is to reduce sugar. At the same time we wish to enjoy our food, and sweetened cereal with milk can be a pleasant and nourishing part of breakfast. The chart "Sugar Content of Some Breakfast Cereals" shows you the percent of sugar in some popular varieties, including the "granola" types. Try some of those with lower sugar content, your old favorites may be among them. For daily use, try to choose from the cereals that contain 25 percent or less total sugar. Some of the cereals with a low sugar content do have a

SUGAR CONTENT OF SOME BREAKFAST CEREALS

Product	Percent of total sugar
Sugar Smacks (K)	56.0
Apple Jacks (K)	54.6
Raisin Bran (GF)	48.0
Sugar Corn Pops (K)	46.0
Super Sugar Crisp (GF)	46.0
Frosted Rice Krinkles (GF)	44.0
Cocoa Krispies (K)	43.0
Cocoa Pebbles (GF)	42.6
Fruity Pebbles (GF)	42.5
Sugar Frosted Flakes of Corn (K)	41.0
Alpha Bits (GF)	38.0
Honey Comb (GF)	37.2
Frosted Rice (K)	37.0
Trix (GM)	35.9
Cocoa Puffs (GM)	33.3
Country Morning (K)	31.0
Golden Grahams (GM)	30.0
Cracklin' Bran (K)	29.0
Raisin Bran (K)	29.0
C.W. Post, raisin (GF)	29.0
Nature Valley Granola Fruit & Nut (GM)	29.0
Frosted Mini Wheats (K)	26.0
Heartland, raisin (P)	26.0
C.W. Post, plain (GF)	25.0
Vita Crunch, regular (OM)	24.0

SUGAR CONTENT OF SOME BREAKFAST CEREALS

Product	Percent of total sugar
Familia (BF)	23.0
Quaker 100% Natural Brown Sugar & Honey (QO)	22.0
Life, cinnamon (QO)	21.0
100% Bran (N)	21.0
All-Bran (K)	19.0
Life (QO)	16.0
Team (N)	14.1
40% Bran (GF)	13.0
Grape Nuts Flakes (GF)	13.3
Product 19 (K)	9.9
Concentrate (K)	9.3
Total (GM)	8.3
Wheaties (GM)	8.2
Rice Krispies (K)	7.8
Grape-Nuts (GF)	7.0
Nutri-Grains (K)	7.0
Special K (K)	5.4
Corn Flakes (K)	5.3
Post Toasties (GF)	5.0
Kix (GM)	4.8
Rice Chex (RP)	4.4
Corn Chex (RP)	4.0
Wheat Chex (RP)	3.5
Cheerios (GM)	3.0
Shredded Wheat (N)	.6
Puffed Wheat (QO)	.5
Puffed Rice (QO)	.1

NOTE: Letters in parentheses following product name indicate manufacturers: General Foods (GF), General Mills (GM), Kellogg (K), Nabisco (N), Quaker Oats (QO), Ralston Purina (RP), Organic Milling (OM), Pet (P).

sweet taste. Adding a little fruit may provide all the sweetening you need.

FAT

✻ I want to eat less fat. How can I do it?

Most Americans eat too much fat, almost one-half of all our calories come from it. That's a lot of fat and you are wise to try to eat less of it. We actually average over 41 percent of our calories as fat. That means that if you usually eat 1,800 calories a day, over 738 of these calories come from fat. One-third less would be a good amount to aim for. Substituting carbohydrate and a little protein for one-third of this fat will benefit you in several ways: not only will you be lowering your calories to help keep your weight at a good level, but you will also be reducing your risk of heart disease and some types of cancer. (Read more about this in Chapters 8 and 9).

Much of the fat you eat you can easily see, like butter, margarine, salad dressing or the visible fat on your steak. A lot of the fat we eat is not so visible. There is invisible fat in the lean portion of meat, in egg yolks, milk, ice cream, olives, peanuts, avocados, walnuts, chocolate cake, pie, and donuts, even soybeans are 17 percent fat. You will have to eat less of both the visible and invisible fats. Trim off all visible fat around your meat, discard skin from poultry, and limit the amount you eat of those foods high in concealed fat.

We add lots of fat when we fry or sauté foods in butter, margarine, oil, lard, or other shortening. When you broil or bake meat, poultry, and fish, the fat cooks off, and if you discard the drippings you end up with less fat than you started with. Try using less fat of all kinds as spreads on breads and rolls and seasonings for vegetables. Flavor can be added with tomatoes and fruit juices, herbs and spices, which are all nearly fat-free. Try a squeeze of lemon and a crushed clove of garlic, for added fat-free flavor. A small amount, one teaspoon or less, of jelly is pleasant on breads and rolls, and if you are eating tasty muffins or biscuits you can skip the spreads entirely. Try it; you can reeducate your taste.

* Exactly what is polyunsaturated fat?

Fats are made up of different fatty acids. These fatty acids are termed *saturated, monounsaturated,* and *polyunsaturated* depending on their chemical structure.

Fats which are made up of saturated fatty acids are solid at room temperature and are found in animal foods like meat, milk, eggs, and cheese. Coconut, chocolate, and palm oil all contain saturated fat and are included in this group. Unsaturated fatty acids may be monounsaturated or polyunsaturated.

Fats made up of unsaturated fatty acids are liquid at room temperature and are found in vegetable foods like corn oil, cottonseed oil, and sunflower oil. The relationship of different types of fat and heart disease is discussed in Chapter 8.

* Which is better for me, butter or margarine?

Butter and margarine are similar to each other in many ways. They look alike, can be used in the same ways in cooking and as a spread, taste somewhat the same, and contain the same number of calories (diet margarine has about one-half the calories of regular margarine or butter because it has some water and air whipped in).

Both butter and margarine are about 80 percent fat. The major difference between the two is the type of fat they contain. Butter is made from cream, contains cholesterol (35 milligrams in one tablespoon), and about 46 percent saturated fat, while margarine is made from vegetable oils (like corn oil margarine—both tube and stick types) and has about 15 percent saturated fat and no cholesterol. Cholesterol is found only in animal fats, *never* in any vegetable oils.

Higher than normal levels of blood cholesterol have been found in many people who have heart attacks. It has been shown that dietary changes—including reduction of cholesterol and also the substitution of polyunsaturated fat for saturated fat—often will lower blood cholesterol levels. This is the reason for using cholesterol-free polyunsaturated margarines in place of butter. (There are other aspects of the relationships of dietary fat to heart disease and these are covered in Chapter 8).

We feel that it is a good idea to lower the total amount of fat you eat—in butter, margarine, and other foods. Unless you have been specifically advised by your physician to use margarine in place of butter, use whichever you prefer, but in limited amounts. Spread either butter or margarine *very lightly* on bread or toast. A good way to get into the habit of using less would be to measure out one-half teaspoon of butter or margarine and spread this on your next slice of toast.

Try using less butter or margarine than usual on potatoes and other vegetables and when cooking or baking. We have found that in most recipes you can reduce the amount of butter called for by one-fourth with little effect on the food. If your favorite special recipe calls for lavish amounts of butter, save it for use on very special occasions.

WATER

* Do I really need to drink water? Don't I get enough liquid in coffee, tea, and other beverages?

Yes, you do need to drink water. Do you realize that your body is over 50 percent water? Everyone knows that their blood contains a large proportion of water, but did you realize that your bones are over 25 percent water? Water is vital to your body's functioning. A person could lose almost all his body fat and over half of his protein and still live, but a loss of as little as one-tenth of your body's weight in water can cause death.

Water is not simply a solvent but is actually part of the body. It lubricates your joints, acts as a cushion for nerves, cools the body, carries essential body substances, removes waste products, and takes part in digestion. It is obvious that water is constantly being used by the body and must be replaced. Water is lost in urine, in the stool, and from the skin and lungs.

Yes, it is true that you may get a large percentage of the water you need from the beverages you usually drink. You also get water from the foods you eat; even bread is about 35 percent water. Additionally, water is formed in the body as a result of the metabolism of food. However, even all of this may not be enough. Generally, you need to replace two to three quarts of water a day to meet your body's requirements. You need at least six cups of fluid each day along with the water you get from food. Subtract the cups of coffee, tea, juice, and milk you drink from six cups. This will tell you how much water you should be drinking each day. For example, if you drink two cups of coffee and one glass of milk you would need three more glasses of water.

When fluid in your body is reduced, thirst is stimulated so you will drink more. For healthy people, this is a good indication of need for more water. You can satisfy this thirst with any beverage you like. Remember, though, that water is the best thirst quencher, it is calorie-free and also may, in certain areas, contain minerals such as calcium, magnesium, zinc, copper, and fluorine.

If you are especially active in warm weather and sweat a lot, it is a good idea to drink a little more water, even after your thirst is satisfied, to be sure that you are replacing the water lost in sweat.

* Should I use bottled water?

Sales of bottled water are skyrocketing. Many people prefer to pay more than a dollar a glass for something they can have, at practically no cost, right from their kitchen faucet. Drinking bottled water has become chic. Advertisements for it stress sophistication as well as the fact that the drink is natural and free of calories. If you wish to pay the price to drink these popular beverages, that should be your choice. You should be aware, however, that if you are using bottled water for supposed health benefits or because it is "purer" than tap water, you are misled.

The U.S. Public Health Drinking Water Standard (1962) established limits on bacterial, physical, radiological, and chemical characteristics of the water supply. These limits are generally accepted by most state and local health agencies.

In most instances this ensures that your drinking water is wholesome and palatable. Occasionally we read that there are high levels of certain pollutants in a specific water supply. The local health department then takes action to improve the water quality.

Bottled water may simply be tap water or water from special wells or springs, but it may be no safer to drink than the water from your kitchen. The mineral content of the bottled waters vary. Some are high in sodium and so should be avoided if you're restricting salt intake. Many bottled waters have small amounts of other minerals like calcium, magnesium, and potassium.

If you drank the leading imported bottled water, you would get a small amount of the minerals you need each day. One liter (a little more than a quart) of Perrier water contains the following minerals: calcium 140.2 mg; magnesium 3.5 mg; sodium 14.0 mg; potassium 1.0 mg.

FIBER

✳ What is fiber?

Fiber is a type of carbohydrate that you cannot digest. It is found in whole grains, fruit, and vegetables. Good sources of fiber are whole-wheat bread, unprocessed bran, grapes, popcorn, beans, and carrots. Regular intake of adequate fiber will promote normal bowel movements.

Fibrous material in meat is protein and can be digested.

✳ Should I add fiber to my diet?

An adequate amount of fiber in the diet is useful in maintaining normal bowel movements and also in helping you to achieve and maintain normal body weight. The other benefits that are claimed for high fiber intake—lowered incidence of colon cancer, diverticulosis, appendicitis, and others—have yet to be proved. While we are waiting for more evidence of fiber's value to our health, it would probably be good for most of us to increase moderately the amount of fiber we eat.

You can do this easily by eating fewer processed foods, for example, eating a whole unpeeled apple instead of applesauce made from peeled apples. Apple cider or juice would have much less fiber than either the whole unpeeled apple or the applesauce. Another way to increase fiber is to use whole-wheat bread, oatmeal, Wheatena, Ralston, shredded wheat. Rye and pumpernickel bread are a combination of whole grains plus white flour, so they too add fiber. (For more information see the highlight box "How to Put More Fiber in Your Diet" and the chart "Dietary Fiber in Foods" in this section.)

When you are buying whole-wheat bread, be sure to check the label to see if whole wheat is first on the list of ingredients. This will tell you that there is more whole-wheat flour in that bread than any other kind of flour. Frequently breads labeled WHEAT are made with mainly white flour and a little caramel coloring added to give the appearance of whole wheat.

HOW TO PUT MORE FIBER IN YOUR DIET

1. Eat more bread made from whole-wheat flour.
2. Use whole grains—cornmeal, brown rice, cracked wheat, barley, rye.
3. Eat hot cereals such as oatmeal, and dry unsugared cereals such as bran flakes, shredded wheat, and oat flakes.
4. Increase your use of fresh fruits and vegetables; use raw and cooked.
5. Eat dried peas and beans—lima beans, kidney beans, split peas, navy beans.
6. Eat less refined sweets—soda, candy, bakery products.

---

* Is bran a good source of fiber?

Some people like to add unprocessed bran to cereals, meat loaves, and other foods to increase their fiber intake. If you wish to do this remember to add very small amounts, one teaspoon to a serving, and gradually increase the amount you use each day to no more than two or three tablespoons. While

Dietary Fiber in Foods

Food	Portion	Grams of dietary fiber*
Apple, unpeeled	1 medium	5.67
Apple, peeled	1 medium	1.96
Banana	1 small	2.08
Baked beans	½ cup	9.27
Bran	1 tablespoon	1.80
Bread, white	1 slice	.68
Bread, whole-wheat	1 slice	2.13
Broccoli, cooked	½ cup	3.18
Cabbage, cooked	½ cup	2.50
Cauliflower, cooked	½ cup	.42
Carrots, cooked	½ cup	2.87
Cereals		
All-Bran	1 ounce	4.00
Corn Flakes	½ cup	1.38
Grape-Nuts	¼ cup	2.10
Shredded Wheat	1 biscuit	3.07
Special K	½ cup	.82
Sugar Puffs	½ cup	.91
Corn, canned	½ cup	4.69
Lettuce	⅙ head	1.53
Peanut butter	1 tablespoon	1.21
Peach, fresh, unpeeled	1	2.28
Pear, unpeeled	1	12.59
Peas, cooked	½ cup	6.67
Strawberries	1 cup	2.65
Tomatoes	1 medium	1.89

* Recommended intakes of dietary fiber are between 30 and 40 grams daily.

a small amount of bran can be beneficial, using too much can irritate your digestive tract, and can cause gas, interfere with normal absorption of minerals, and even, in extreme cases, form an impaction in your intestine. Moderation is the key here as it is with many other things.

If you are not sure that you need the additional fiber supplied by bran, there is a simple guide: if your stool floats, it is an indication that it has sufficient bulk and that you are eating enough fiber. The muffin recipes at the end of this chapter are a good way to add fiber to your diet.

SPECIAL MUFFIN RECIPES

We like muffins. They are delicious, simple to make, economical (a regular corn muffin costs 30 to 45 cents—ours cost 7 cents), an easy way to introduce whole grains and fiber into your diet, and easy to freeze (bake once and have muffins for a week).

Even if you do not bake, look over the following recipes and you may be tempted to try at least one of them. Our preparation technique, the "muffin method," is so simple and quick, anyone can turn out a delicious product. From the time you walk into your kitchen, till you enjoy your first bite of a warm muffin, should not take more than a half hour.

We have eliminated salt in every recipe and cut down on fat and sugar whenever possible, while at the same time producing a delicious muffin. Using cupcake papers reduces cleanup and eliminates the oil or shortening used to grease the pan, which cuts down on calories and fat; spray shortening products (like Pam) may be used to "grease" the muffin tin. We like big muffins, so we fill our muffin tins to the rim and get eight to ten muffins per recipe. If you'd prefer smaller ones, fill the muffin tin two-thirds full, and the recipe will yield ten to twelve medium-size muffins. Note the special instructions for modified diets at the end of the recipes.

Oatmeal-Yogurt Muffins
Yield: 8 large muffins

   1 cup plain low-fat yogurt
  ¼ cup oil
   1 egg
1¼ cups flour
  ¾ cup quick-cooking rolled oats
   2 tablespoons sugar
   2 teaspoons baking powder
  ¼ teaspoon baking soda

Preheat oven to 400°F.

Grease muffin tins lightly or line with cupcake papers.

In a 2-cup measuring cup, measure yogurt and oil; add egg; stir to combine.

In a bowl combine remaining dry ingredients.

Add yogurt mixture to flour mixture, stirring approximately 25 strokes.

Fill muffin tins to the rim.

Bake for 20 minutes.

> HINT: 1 cup of skim milk may be substituted for the yogurt, also omit ¼ teaspoon baking soda; this change reduces the sodium to 116 mg. sodium per muffin, or 23 mg. sodium when using low-sodium baking powder. Using skim milk will give the muffin a slightly different taste.
>
> Per muffin: 166 calories; 147 mg. sodium or 54.5 mg. sodium using low-sodium baking powder

Corn Muffins
Yield: 8 large muffins

1 cup skim milk
3 tablespoons oil
1 egg
1 cup flour
1 cup yellow cornmeal
¼ cup sugar
1 tablespoon baking powder

Preheat oven to 400°F.

Grease muffin tin lightly or line with cupcake papers.

In a 2-cup measuring cup, measure milk and oil; add egg; stir to combine.

In a bowl combine remaining dry ingredients.

Add milk mixture to flour mixture, stirring approximately 25 strokes.

Fill muffin tins to the rim.

Bake for 20 minutes.

HINT: To vary flavor add 1 teaspoon grated lemon rind and ½ teaspoon lemon juice. Delicious!
Per muffin: 196 calories; 161 mg. sodium or 22 mg. sodium using low-sodium baking powder

Whole Wheat–Corn Muffins
Yield: 8 large muffins

1¼ cups skim milk
½ cup honey
¼ cup oil
1 egg
1 cup whole-wheat flour
1 cup cornmeal
4 teaspoons baking powder

Preheat oven to 400°F.
Grease muffin tin lightly or line with cupcake papers.
In a 2-cup measuring cup, measure milk, honey, and oil; add egg; stir to combine.
In a bowl combine remaining dry ingredients.
Add milk mixture to flour mixture, stirring approximately 25 strokes.
Fill muffin tins to the rim.
Bake for 20 minutes.

Per muffin: 247 calories; 215 mg. sodium or 30 mg. sodium using low-sodium baking powder

Rice Muffins
Yield: 8 large muffins

1 cup skim milk
2 tablespoons oil
1 egg
1 cup flour
½ cup whole-wheat flour
1 cup cooked brown rice
2 tablespoons sugar
2 teaspoons baking powder

Preheat oven to 400°F.

Grease muffin tins lightly or line with cupcake papers.

In a 2-cup measuring cup, measure milk; add oil and egg; stir to combine.

In a bowl combine remaining dry ingredients.

Add milk mixture to flour mixture, stirring about 25 strokes.

Fill muffin tins to the rim.

Bake for 20 minutes.

> HINT: 1 cup of cooked regular white rice may be substituted for brown rice. *Do not use instant rice.*
>
> Per muffin: 193 calories; 116 mg. sodium or 23 mg. sodium using low sodium baking powder

Bran Muffins
Yield: 10 large muffins

1⅓ cups skim milk
⅓ cup honey
2 tablespoons oil
1 egg
1½ cups whole-wheat flour
½ cup flour
1 cup raisin-bran cereal
1 tablespoon baking powder
½ teaspoon baking soda

Preheat oven to 400°F.

Grease muffin tins lightly or line with cupcake papers.

In a 2-cup measuring cup, measure milk and honey; add oil and egg; stir to combine.

In a bowl combine remaining dry ingredients.

Add milk mixture to flour mixture, stirring about 25 strokes.

Fill muffins to the rim.

Bake for 20 minutes.

> HINT: To make this recipe with unprocessed bran, substitute ⅓ cup unprocessed bran and ¼ cup raisins for 1 cup Raisin Bran cereal.
>
> Per muffin: 174 calories; 239 mg. sodium or 128 mg. sodium using low sodium baking powder

Apple Muffins
Yield: 8 large muffins

1 cup skim milk
2 tablespoons oil
2 tablespoons honey
1 egg
1½ cups flour
½ cup whole-wheat flour
¼ cup brown sugar
2 teaspoons baking powder
1 teaspoon cinnamon
1 large apple, pared, seeded, and grated

Preheat oven to 400°F.

Grease muffin tin lightly or line with cupcake papers.

In a 2-cup measuring cup, measure milk; add oil, honey, and egg; stir to combine.

In a bowl combine remaining dry ingredients.

Add milk mixture to flour mixture, stirring approximately 25 strokes.

Fill muffin tins to the rim.

Bake for 20 minutes.

> NOTE: This is a sweet muffin and makes a good substitute for cake.
> Per muffin: 181 calories; 116 mg. sodium or 24 mg. sodium using low-sodium baking powder

Buckwheat-Banana Muffins
Yield: 10 large muffins

¾ cup skim milk
¼ cup honey
2 tablespoons oil
1 egg
1 cup white flour
½ cup whole-wheat flour
2 teaspoons baking soda
½ cup buckwheat groats (kasha)
1 ripe banana, peeled and mashed

Preheat oven to 400°F.

Grease muffin tin lightly or line with cupcake papers.

In a 2-cup measuring cup, measure milk and honey; add oil and egg; stir to combine.

In a bowl combine remaining dry ingredients except for banana.

Add milk mixture and banana to flour mixture, stirring approximately 25 strokes.

Fill muffin tins to the rim.

Bake for 20 minutes.

> NOTE: The flavor of these muffins mellows so that you find they are even more delicious the second and third day.
> Per muffin: 168 calories; 215 mg. sodium

Variations

Any recipe may be varied by adding one or a combination of any of these ingredients:

⅓ cup blueberries
¼ cup raisins
¼ cup chopped dates
¼ cup chopped prunes
¼ cup chopped apricots
½ cup chopped fresh cherries
¼ cup chopped fresh cranberries
¼ cup chopped nuts
¼ cup chopped figs

Storage

The muffins will stay fresh for two to three days if you store them in a closed plastic bag on the kitchen counter (refrigerating them accelerates staling). For longer storage, freeze in a closed plastic bag. Remove muffins one or a few at a time. They freeze well and may be kept in the freezer four to six weeks.

Reheating

Muffins may be reheated at 325°F for 5 minutes. If frozen, heat at 300°F for 10 to 12 minutes. For an interesting breakfast treat, before reheating, slice a muffin in half and insert a piece of your favorite cheese, now heat for 5 minutes. Combine your cheese muffin with juice and coffee and you'll have a quick, nutritious, and good-tasting breakfast.

Modified Diets

On a special diet? If so, you can still enjoy these muffins.

Low cholesterol: Substitute 2 egg whites for 1 whole egg. Use only corn, safflower, cottonseed, soybean, or sunflower oil.

Low sodium: We have eliminated salt in all recipes but to reduce sodium even further be sure to use low-sodium baking powder. Cellu is a widely available brand or see Chapter 8's salt and sodium section, for a recipe for low-sodium baking powder you can prepare yourself.

Avoid those recipes calling for *baking soda*, except for the Oatmeal-Yogurt Muffins recipe which is especially modified for you. (See Hint at bottom of recipe.) One teaspoon of baking soda has 1000 mg. of sodium and there is no available substitute.

Diabetic: When you make the muffin recipes, fill each muffin tin only two-thirds full. This will give you a medium rather than a large muffin. For all the recipes, 1 medium muffin may be used in your daily meal plan as 2 bread exchanges plus 1 fat exchange. The Whole Wheat–Corn Muffins is the only recipe you should avoid.

2

More Nutrients:
How Much Is Enough?

Almost one-third of all adult Americans take vitamins regularly. When questioned, 80 percent of the people said they believe they could get all their vitamins and minerals from a balanced diet, but these same people did not believe their diet was balanced.

Sales of vitamin and mineral supplements are $1.2 billion annually and still growing. By 1988, $3.5 billion will be spent on these supplements—a startling increase even though one-half of the figure will be due to price increases.

Are we really in need of these supplements? Isn't it true that we can get all the nutrients we need if we eat a varied, balanced diet? Are some of our common problems of aches, pains, graying hair, colds, dental disease and loss of taste related to marginal nutrient deficiencies?

To answer those questions, we have to consider not only what we know about nutrients and our need for them, but also the things that we all do, more or less, that affect our nutrition:

- We aren't very active, so we really need less food (less calories anyway).

- We eat mostly refined and processed foods (even freezing is processing).

- We are often dieting to lose weight (some of us attempt this every once in a while—others more often).

- We eat food high in calories from fats and sugars (low in other nutrients).

- Many of our foods have lost some of their original value because of poor handling (during shipping, storage, cooking).

- We are subjected to stresses that may increase our need for nutrients (illness, surgery, medications, smoking, alcohol, or even air pollution).

In view of all these, it seems that we may be short of certain nutrients, so wouldn't it be best if we all took some vitamins and minerals just to be on the safe side? To that question we must answer a guarded "maybe." It certainly wouldn't hurt for you to take a mulivitamin-mineral supplement, *once daily*, that contains Recommended Dietary Allowance (RDA) levels of required vitamins and minerals, for insurance. There are some problems with this approach. It might give you a false sense of security so that you will give less thought to what you eat. You might be tempted on certain days when you are not feeling up to par to take an additional dose. Vitamins and minerals are not things where a little more is always better. In fact, a little more, in the case of some vitamins and minerals, can be a lot worse.

We have given considerable study and thought to the ways people meet their nutrient needs. We have liberalized our ideas in the last few years; we are no longer adamantly opposed to supplementation. We recognize that supplementation is appropriate and even necessary in some situations. But, on the other hand, we feel bound to restrain the overenthusiastic user.

What we have attempted to do in this chapter is to give you a grasp of the complexities and issues involved. We do not have all the answers. However, after reading what *we do know* you will be better able to decide for yourself.

* How do I know if the "research" I read about is accurate?

One important point to keep in mind when you read information on vitamin and mineral needs is that there is a vast difference between scientific and anecdotal evidence. Anecdotal evidence is merely observation of a happening. It can only show that more study is warranted. For example: A woman reported in a popular magazine that she had cured her leukemia by drinking carrot juice. This might call for further investigation but surely does not constitute proof that carrot juice cures leukemia.

On the other hand, a scientific experiment has an adequate number of subjects, can be replicated by another investigator, and has had the results carefully evaluated. We often question research and seek further evidence. You should also.

Read testimonials cautiously, think of research as *some* evidence that should be considered, and then make a decision for yourself tempered with a good dose of common sense.

VITAMINS

* Why do I need vitamins? What are they?

Vitamins are substances made by plants and animals and used in our bodies' metabolism. In a word, they are regulators. Although we need only small amounts of vitamins we either can't make them or we don't make enough, and so we must get them from the foods we eat. Each vitamin is different from the others in its chemical structure and also in the way it works. See the chart "Vitamin Sources" later in this section.

Some vitamins are usually known by letters A, C, D, and so on, while others are more commonly known by their chemical names, such as thiamine and riboflavin.

* Are natural vitamins better than synthetic ones?

Synthetic vitamins are identical in every way to their natural counterparts. Your body cannot tell the difference. They are utilized in the same way whether they were made in a laboratory or extracted from an animal or plant. When vitamin B_{12} was isolated from liver, it took 1 ton of fresh liver to produce 20 milligrams of the vitamin. Fortunately, since 1973, vitamin B_{12} has been synthesized in the laboratory.

Rose hips supplement, touted as an excellent source of vitamin C, actually contains very little (2 percent). Tablets containing rose hips as the only source of vitamin C would be too large to swallow. When you see *Rose Hips Vitamin C* on a label you are getting only a tiny amount from the rose hips and most from another source of vitamin C, usually a synthetic form.

Beware of the terms "natural" and "organic" on vitamin labels. As there is no legal definition for these terms, they can be used freely. (See the first question in Chapter 3, "Are natural foods best?") You may choose to use these "natural" supplements anyway for other reasons.

Some people object to the fact that many nutrient supplements contain synthetic emulsifiers, waxes, saccharin, sugar, and artificial colors. Some natural brands do not. Be sure to read the labels carefully, since additives may be in natural vitamins as well. What generally separates natural and synthetic vitamins is cost—natural being more expensive. Paying more does not ensure that one type is better than another. Remember, your body can't tell the difference.

* How are nutrients measured?

It's easy to be confused by all the different terms that are used to measure nutrients. Even a simple term like *calorie*— Oh, everyone knows what a calorie is, you're thinking, that's what makes you fat. But actually a calorie (really a *kilocalorie**) is merely the amount of heat needed to raise the temperature of a little more than a quart of water 1 degree Centigrade.

Heat and energy are the same thing (about 80 percent of the calories or energy in food makes heat, and the remainder provides the energy to run our bodies). So calories equal heat

---

* There is interest in substituting the term *kilojoule* for *kilocalorie* to measure the energy in food. To change Calories to kilojoules, you multiply by 4.2. That way an 80 Calorie apple would be 336 joules. A 1,200 Calorie diet may be easier to stick to if you think of it as 5,040 joules.

equal energy. Keep that in mind, the next time you read an ad that says "Krispie Krunchies are loaded with energy but low in calories."

Fat, protein, and carbohydrates are often measured in grams (the metric unit of weight). To help you visualize this, one small apple weighs about 100 grams and one level teaspoon of salt weighs 5 grams.

Vitamins and minerals are often measured in milligrams (mg.) and micrograms (mcg.). There are 1,000 milligrams in a gram and 1,000 micrograms in a milligram. In other words, a microgram is one-millionth of a gram. So when we speak of our daily need for 3 micrograms of vitamin B_{12}, that is a minute amount.

If all these measurements are not confusing enough, there is more! Some vitamins are measured in international units (I.U.). An *international unit* is a measure of biological activity. It is the amount of that nutrient that relieves deficiency symptoms in a laboratory rat. It is a different amount for different vitamins. Vitamin A is also measured as retinol equivalents (RE). (See the question "I sometimes see vitamin A listed as RE . . ." in the Vitamin A section of this chapter.) Vitamin D is measured in I.U. or milligrams (40 I.U. equal 1 milligram). Vitamin E is measured in I.U. or milligram alpha-tocopherol equivalents (αTE), the most active form of the vitamin.

✳ What is the RDA?

The amount of vitamins that a person needs depends on many things. Age, sex, size, state of health or disease, activity, and environment affect vitamin requirements.

We are often asked how much of a specific vitamin a person should have. That is difficult to answer because each person is an individual and so it follows that their nutrient needs are individual too. There is no way that we predict precisely how much of a nutrient one person needs. There is, however, a guide.

The Food and Nutrition Board of the National Academy of Sciences has a committe on dietary allowances. This committee establishes "recommendations for the average daily amounts of nutrients that *population groups* should consume over a period of time." These are called the "Recommended Dietary Allowances" (RDA), not to be confused with the U.S. RDA (see the following question). The recommendations are not requirements for individuals, but are planned to meet the needs of groups of healthy people over a period of time. That's why for all nutrients listed, except for calories, recommendations are greater than most healthy individuals require. This means that you don't have to take in daily all the quantities listed for each nutrient in order to be well nourished.

We feel, however, that it's a good idea for anyone who is interested enough in nutrition to be reading this book to know what the RDA is. It is often referred to in newspaper or magazine articles.

* What is the U.S. RDA?

The U.S. RDA is the United States Recommended Daily Allowances. They were developed to be used on food labels

Nutrition Information per Serving
Serving Size: 1 ounce

	1 ounce cereal	With ½ cup vitamin D fortified whole milk
Calories	100	180
Protein	3 g.	7 g.
Carbohydrate	23 g.	29 g.
Fat	1 g.	5 g.
Sodium	195 mg.	255 mg.

Percentages of U.S. Recommended Daily Allowances (U.S. RDA)

Protein	6%	10%
Vitamin A	25%	30%
Vitamin C	*	*
Thiamine	25%	30%

* Contains less than 2% of the U.S. RDA of these nutrients.

and in most cases they are the highest RDA for each nutrient suggested for any age-sex group (see typical cereal label on page 34).

The U.S. RDA replaces the Minimum Daily Requirement (MDR) you have seen on cereal and vitamin labels for years.

Because Recommended Dietary Allowances is too cumbersome to be used on a label, the U.S. RDA is a simplification that will fit. Nutrient values of foods are often given as percentages of the U.S. RDA.

From this you can tell that the cereal alone provides 25 percent of the U.S. RDA for vitamin A and thiamine with lesser amounts of other nutrients.

* Can large amounts of vitamins be dangerous?

A woman who was taking large amounts of vitamin A for several years for a chronic skin condition developed headaches, stiff muscles, and an enlarged liver. She was being poisoned by the excess quantity of vitamin A that was stored in her body. This condition is called "hypervitaminosis."

An excess of any vitamin in the body is termed *hypervitaminosis*. This will most likely occur with the overuse of vitamins A and D. Because you can store vitamins A and D in the liver, excess amounts of these can accumulate and cause ill effects. This is an example of *too much* of a good thing.

Hypervitaminosis has developed in adults who have taken 5,000 RE (25,000 I.U.) of vitamin A for a long time. It is best to limit supplements of this vitamin to no more than 3,000 RE (15,000 I.U.) daily.

* How long can I keep vitamins without their losing their potency?

Vitamins usually remain stable for four or five years. Many brands have an expiration date on their labels and that can be your guide. If there is no expiration date, it's a good idea to date the container yourself so you'll know how long you've had them.

Using vitamins after their expiration date is not dangerous, but you may not be getting any benefit from them, because they have reduced potency. A rule of thumb is that if there is any change in color, taste, smell, or appearance you should discard them. Vitamins in capsules last longer than the pressed tablets (those are the ones that look like aspirins).

Store vitamins in their original containers, in a cool, dry place. The kitchen and bathroom, where you usually find the vitamin bottles, are not the best place for them. The heat and humidity hastens deterioration. A shelf in your linen closet or on the top of your dresser is a better place to keep vitamins than on the kitchen table.

If you buy vitamins in bulk amounts, keep a large supply in the refrigerator. Remove a small supply to another container and store as suggested above.

VITAMIN SOURCES

Vitamin	Source	RDA	U.S. RDA
A	Liver, butter, margarine, milk, eggs, yellow vegetables and fruits, dark green leafy vegetables	1,000 mcg. RE (males) 800 mcg. RE (females)	5000 I.U.*
D	Fortified milk, margarine, butter, liver (exposure to sunlight)	5 mcg.	400 I.U.*
E	Cereals, wheat germ, nuts, legumes, vegetable oil	10.0 mg. αTE (males) 8.0 mg. αTE (females)	30 I.U.*
K	Spinach, cauliflower, cabbage, liver	70–140 mcg.†	

Vitamin Sources

Vitamin	Source	RDA	U.S. RDA
C	Citrus fruits, tomatoes, cabbage, cantaloupe, broccoli, strawberries, potatoes	60.0 mg.	60.0 mg.
B_1 (thiamine)	Whole-grain cereals, breads, enriched cereals and breads, liver, pork, wheat germ, brewer's yeast, peanuts, milk	1.4 mg. (males) 1.0 mg. (females)	1.5 mg.
B_2 (riboflavin)	Milk, organ meats, eggs, green leafy vegetables, yeast, peas, beans	1.6 mg. (males) 1.2 mg. (females)	1.7 mg.
Niacin	Lean meat, fish, poultry, liver, kidney, whole-grain cereals and bread, enriched cereals and bread, peanuts, yeast	18.0 mg. (males) 13.0 mg. (females)	20.0 mg.
Folic acid	Green leafy vegetables, oranges, liver, kidney, yeast	0.4 mg.	0.4 mg.
B_6	Meat, liver, wheat germ, peanuts, corn, whole-grain cereals and breads, milk	2.2 mg. (males) 2.0 mg. (females)	2.0 mg.
B_{12}	Milk, poultry, fish	3 mcg.	6 mcg.
Biotin	Liver, sweetbreads, yeast, eggs, dried peas and beans	0.10–0.20 mg.	0.30 mg.†

VITAMIN SOURCES

Vitamin	*Source*	*RDA*	*U.S. RDA*
Pantothenic acid	Liver, yeast, eggs, peanuts, whole-grain cereals and breads, beef, tomatoes, broccoli, salmon	4.0–7.0 mg.	10.0 mg.†

* For some nutrients, different methods of measurement are used in RDA and U.S. RDA.

† These nutrients are not found in main table of RDA because there is less information about them, so a range of estimated safe and adequate daily dietary intake is provided rather than specific recommendations.

* How much of the vitamins and minerals in food is lost during cooking?

Cooking does destroy nutrients, but before you switch to a raw food diet keep in mind that cooking has advantages as well. It softens fiber and cellulose releasing trapped nutrients, destroys natural toxic substances found in some foods (like cabbage and soybeans), and makes foods palatable.

Water-soluble vitamins (the B family and C) and minerals are most likely to be lost during cooking. The vitamins are destroyed by heat and leach into the cooking water. Minerals find their way into the cooking water as well but are generally heat stable.

Keep that water! Vegetable liquid is a good source of vitamins and minerals—use it to make gravy, soup, or the base for a stew. When a package says "add water," add your vegetable liquid instead. Use it to reconstitute mashed potatoes or as the liquid to cook rice. It will add both nutrients and flavor.

Pressure cooking and steaming will reduce nutrient loss and should be used in place of boiling when possible. The amount of vitamins destroyed in cooking is hard to tell. Nutrient loss occurs in storage, handling, and finally in cooking. Below are ranges of loss that can be expected. The longer the cooking time the greater the loss.

Vitamin	Percent of loss in cooking
A	0–40
D	0–25
C	0–100
Thiamine*	0–80
Riboflavin	0–75
Niacin	0–75
B_6	0–40
B_{12}	0–30
Folacin†	0–100

* Toasting a slice of bread for 30 to 70 seconds destroys 10 to 30 percent.

† Storing vegetables at room temperature results in up to 70 percent loss in three days.

Vitamin A

* I sometimes see vitamin A listed as RE. What does that mean?

You may be confused by the fact that sometimes you see vitamin A measured in international units (I.U.) while at other times it is given as retinol equivalents (RE). Retinol is the chemical name for vitamin A. However, the body gets vitamin A either as retinol or as carotene. Carotene is not as potent a source of vitamin A as the retinol form. The newer term "retinol equivalents" is more acurate and you will be seeing vitamin A measured as RE in the future. (See chart "Vitamin Sources" to the RDA for vitamin A.)

* Will vitamin A help me to see in the dark?

Taking extra vitamin A will not help you find seats more easily in a dim theater, but you do need vitamin A for normal night vision. It is part of the substance that helps your eyes adjust to the dark. A vitamin supplement would be beneficial only if you were deficient in this nutrient.

* I have heard that vitamin A can prevent cancer. Is it true?

Recent studies show that the risk of cancer is less when a person eats foods rich in vitamin A and *carotene* (a yellow pigment that is changed into vitamin A in the body). This was found to be true even among cigarette smokers who have a greater risk of lung cancer.

Vitamin A is found in eggs, liver, and whole milk. It is dissolved in the fat in these foods and that is why skim milk, milk that has had most of the fat removed, has a large portion of the vitamin A removed as well. To compensate for this, most skim milk that you buy has had vitamin A added. The result is that it is a better source of this nutrient than whole milk (one cup skim milk gives 500 I.U.; one cup whole milk gives 300 I.U.).

Carotene is the coloring that gives carrots their bright orange-yellow hue. It does the same for sweet potatoes, winter squash, peaches, and pumpkin. There is carotene in green vegetables too, but its color is masked by the dark green chlorophyll. Carotene is also used as a food color, giving a rich golden glow to margarine, cheese, cereal, and cake mixes.

The usual advice given to ensure enough vitamin A is to eat a bright yellow or deep green leafy vegetable at least every other day. In view of the evidence that this nutrient might be protective against cancer, it is probably a better idea to eat one or two servings of carotene-rich vegetables every day. (See the question "Since I began eating vegetarian meals the palms of my hands have yellowed. . . ." Chapter 10.)

* Is every yellow and green vegetable or fruit a good source of carotene?

Many deep yellow fruits (apricots, peaches, cantaloupe) and vegetables (carrots, sweet potatoes, winter squash), deep green leafy and stem vegetables (spinach, beet greens, collards, asparagus, broccoli) are rich in carotenes that your body can convert into vitamin A. The deeper green leaves are richer sources than the pale green leaves of lettuce and cabbage. Not every yellow fruit or vegetable is a good source of carotenes. Corn, pears, and summer squash get some of their color from pigments that are not sources of vitamin A. (For best sources, see the chart "Vitamin A Content of Some Foods.")

Vitamin A Content of Some Foods

Food	Portion	I.U.	RE
Sweet potato, baked	1 medium	9,230	1,846
Spinach, cooked	½ cup	7,290	1,458
Carrots, diced, cooked	½ cup	7,110	1,422
Collards, cooked	½ cup	5,130	1,026
Broccoli, cooked	1 stalk	4,500	900
Cantaloupe	⅛	2,310	462
Peach	1 medium	1,330	266
Apricot	1 medium	963	193
Lettuce	¼ head	450	90
Summer squash, diced	½ cup	410	82
Yellow corn*, canned	½ cup	345	69
Wax beans, canned	½ cup	70	14
Cabbage, shredded	½ cup	45	9
Bartlett pear	1 medium	30	6

* White corn contains little vitamin A.

Vitamin D

✳ I have heard that too much vitamin D is dangerous. Is that true?

Vitamin D is usually measured in I.U. or international units. You may also see it given as micrograms. One microgram is equal to 40 I.U.

The Recommended Dietary Allowance of vitamin D for adults is 5 micrograms daily (still commonly referred to as 200 I.U.). As little as five times that amount taken for a long time causes dangerous calcium deposits in the kidney. Large amounts, 150,000 I.U. (3,750 micrograms), are taken daily for treatment of arthritis. In a short period this has caused calcification of the kidneys and other organs, loss of appetite, and disturbances in vision. Vitamin D has not been shown to help arthritis.

Because of the danger of toxicity from amounts of vitamin D that are close to required amounts, it is wise for you not to take more than 2,000 I.U. (50 micrograms) a day from food and supplements combined. Remember, many multivitamin preparations contain 400 I.U. of vitamin D in a single capsule.

* If vitamin D is the sunshine vitamin, can I get all I need from the sun?

It is true that when you are outdoors, the ultraviolet rays in sunlight act on a substance in your skin called 7-dehydrocholestrerol and change it to vitamin D. That's why this vitamin has been called the "sunshine vitamin." It really isn't a good idea for most of us to depend on this source alone. The reason for this is that smog and dust in the atmosphere can screen out the special rays of sunlight that make vitamin D. Clothing keeps the sun's rays from the skin as does dark skin, which can keep as much as 95 percent of the sun's rays from penetrating. Even ordinary windowpanes prevent the rays from reaching us. As we age, our skin has a more difficult time making vitamin D. Sunlight is not enough—we need other sources.

Foods that contain a little vitamin D are egg yolk, liver, and some fish, but unfortified foods are really not good sources. Fortunately almost all milk sold, fresh, canned, or dry, has been fortified with vitamin D. Two cups of vitamin D fortified milk provide 200 I.U. (or 5 micrograms), the Recommended Dietary Allowance for adults.

Sometimes you will notice that vitamin D has been added to other foods like ready-to-eat cereals, milk flavorings, and breakfast/snack bars. This additional source of vitamin D is not necessary and may be harmful. (See preceding question.)

Cod liver oil is a very rich source of vitamin D but really should be considered as a supplement not a food. One tablespoon has 30 micrograms of vitamin D.

* I read that vitamin D is really a hormone. Isn't it a vitamin?

Vitamin D has been grouped along with the vitamins since its isolation in 1931. It really is more like a hormone in that it is formed in one organ and acts on other tissues in the body. Vitamin D, either taken in food or made in the skin, is converted to its active form, a hormone, in the liver and kidneys. After its conversion, it is called "calcitriol." It is used by the body to aid the absorption and excretion of minerals, calcium, and phosphorus. It also has a role in bone formation. If the kidney is diseased so that it cannot convert vitamin D to its hormone form, calcitriol (Rocaltrol) can be given.

Vitamin E

* I have had painful leg cramps since I was forty. Will vitamin E help?

There is a good chance it might. Vitamin E seems to improve blood circulation. Four hundred I.U. daily for three months relieved calf pains caused by poor circulation. This was found in a double blind study (where neither the subjects nor the observers knew who was really taking the vitamin E), so the results were not due to placebo effect. In fact, the improvement was shown to be in proportion to the increased amount of vitamin E in the muscles. Those treated with vitamin E had improved circulation in their legs. Night leg cramps are also relieved with a similar supplement. (See chart "Vitamin Sources" for the RDA for vitamin E.)

* Can vitamin E be used to slow down aging?

Nobody really knows. Because vitamin E acts as an antioxidant some people believe that it can be used to counteract the aging of our body cells. We are all constantly being bombarded with atmospheric radiation. This radiation damages our cells in several ways, producing so-called aging pigment that is like a rust spot. One theory is that if we have enough vitamin E, it will slow down this destruction.

Adult mice were given large doses of vitamin E to study its effect on aging. The dose of vitamin E they took would be equal to your taking about 2,000 I.U. (or milligrams) daily. After one year the mice had no improvement in their body organs and no reduction in death rate. One positive note was that the mice had less of the aging pigment in their cells.

It is very difficult to test the theory out in people because it takes them much longer to age. So rather than waiting for some proof that vitamin E slows down aging, some poeple are taking it early "just in case it should prove to be true." Even if it doesn't help, it probably won't cause harm. Supplements of up to 800 I.U. daily for over three years were not toxic.

* Will vitamin E help to protect me from air pollution?

It might be helpful. Large amounts of vitamin E given to rats helped protect their lungs from the bad effects of two substances commonly found in polluted air—ozone and nitrogen dioxide. These results may be applicable to us because our lungs are damaged by the same pollutants.

* Is vitamin E a "wonder" nutrient?

From the preceding questions it may appear that vitamin E is a wonder nutrient that can be helpful for many ailments. Unfortunately, this is not the case. Except for its use in the specific situations discussed and perhaps in the case of cystic breast disease and menopause discomfort (see Chapter 5) vitamin E has not been shown to be a cure-all. In fact, it has been found to be useless as a supplement to improve athletic ability, or in treating sexual performance, muscular dystrophies, skin diseases, sterility, ulcers, cancer, and heart disease. The list could be much longer.

Much research is underway at this time to find additional uses for the vitamin. But until these uses are shown to be effective under controlled experimental conditions, they should not be relied on and most certainly should not take the place of appropriate medical diagnosis and treatment.

Vitamin K

* Why is there no vitamin K in my multivitamin supplement?

It's very unlikely that you would be deficient in vitamin K, the vitamin needed for normal blood clotting. You get half of the vitamin K you need from food—green leafy vegetables mainly—the other half is made by the bacteria that live in your intestine. Because you have these two sources, it is unusual to become deficient. That is one reason why vitamin K is not included in multivitamin supplements. Neither is it added to foods (infant formula is an exception). Another reason is that the synthetic forms of the vitamin are toxic in large doses and available only by prescription.

Vitamin C

* I am confused about what I read in the newspaper. Will vitamin C help to prevent colds?

People often tell us that since they take 1 gram or so of vitamin C each day (see Chart "Vitamin Sources" for the RDA for vitamin C), they do not get as many colds as they used to. This type of reporting is called "anecdotal" and results like this cannot be taken seriously. Reliable information is obtained from controlled studies that are subjected to scientific scrutiny, and even these are complicated by the facts that colds are caused by a variety of viruses and the researchers must depend on how well their subjects can diagnose the cold and describe it.

It appears from some studies that vitamin C does slightly reduce the possiblity of catching a cold and also that the vitamin acts as an antihistamine and so may reduce cold symptoms. You have to weigh these slight benefits against the risks of taking continued large doses of vitamin C.

While many people have taken large amounts of vitamin C for a long time without any apparent ill effects, large amounts of C increase the outputs of both oxalic acid and uric acid in the urine. These substances are components of kidney stones so they may increase your risk of forming them. Also it has been shown that when you take large amounts of vitamin C for a long time, your body begins to use it up faster, you become dependent on large amounts, so that if you abruptly reduce your intake you may become deficient. Massive doses of vitamin C cause diarrhea as much of the dose is not absorbed and so draws water into the intestine. It is not a good idea for diabetics who test their urine routinely to take large amounts of vitamin C. It can cause false-negative results with Tes-Tape, Clinistix and Dextrostix, and false-positive results with Clinitest drops. Large amounts of C may invalidate the laboratory test for blood in the stool so that potentially serious illnesses may be overlooked.

* Do I need extra vitamin C if I smoke?

Recent studies show that smokers had a higher turnover of vitamin C in their bodies. They needed to take in at least 40 milligrams of vitamin C daily in order for them to maintain adequate body levels of the vitamin. This amount is more than twice the Recommended Dietary Allowance for adults. If you smoke, you should be sure to eat two servings of vitamin C–rich foods daily. Taking in extra vitamin C may be a problem for smokers. The extra C will acidify the urine and as nicotine is excreted more rapidly in an acidic urine, the smoker might have an increased desire for cigarettes.

* Does stress increase my need for vitamin C?

In certain situations, the body may use up larger than normal amounts of vitamin C. Infections and fevers have been shown to deplete tissue levels of the vitamin as does other stress, such as injury, shock, illness, surgery, and bone fractures. Even psychological stress may increase your need for vitamin C. There is no agreement on just how much additional vitamin C is needed in stress situations, but often 1 to 2 grams, which is ten or so times the usual requirement, is given.

Supplementation at this level is becoming increasingly popular. We are not convinced of the desirability; however, neither do we feel it is harmful. Scientific evidence has not shown any risk from continued supplements in these amounts.

SOURCES OF VITAMIN C

Food	Portion	Milligrams of vitamin C	Calories
Bean sprouts, mung	½ cup	10	21
Broccoli	½ cup	53	26
Brussels sprouts	½ cup	63	70
Cabbage	½ cup	17	12
Cantaloupe	¼	45	30
Grapefruit	½	44	40
Green pepper	½	47	11
Lemonade	1 cup	17	100
Orange juice, fresh	½ cup	62	55
Orange juice, canned	½ cup	50	57
Orange juice, frozen	½ cup	60	56
Potato, baked	1 medium	31	95
Potato, boiled	1 medium	22	76
Potato, instant mashed	½ cup	6	83
Potato chips	10	3	113
Strawberries	½ cup	44	28
Sweet potato, baked	1 medium	25	141
Tangerine	1 medium	27	46
Tomato juice	½ cup	19	23
Tomato soup	1 cup	15	104
Watermelon	1 slice	30	115

Vitamin B_2

* Will taking riboflavin (vitamin B_2) help to prevent cataracts?

Rats fed diets deficient in riboflavin (vitamin B_2) can develop cataracts (corneal opacities) and other eye disorders. That is why you may have heard that taking riboflavin will prevent cataracts.

In man, a deficiency of riboflavin causes extra blood vessels to develop in the cornea of the eye along with burning, itching, and tearing. Cataracts, however, have never been linked to a riboflavin deficiency. If a person eating a diet low in riboflavin had some eye symptoms that are known to be related to riboflavin deficiency, taking 2 milligrams of riboflavin (more than the amount needed daily) would relieve the symptoms. Taking extra riboflavin would not make the eyes "healthier."

You are not likely to have a riboflavin deficiency, as this vitamin is widely distributed in foods. Milk, cheese, organ meats, other meat, fish, and leafy green vegetables are good sources. Whole-grain cereals and breads and enriched cereals and breads also contain some riboflavin.

Vitamin B_{12}

* How can I be sure that I am getting all the vitamin B_{12} I need each day?

You really don't need a source of B_{12} every day. You have vitamin B_{12} stored in your body and it would take years to use it up. You probably have a three- to five-year supply stored in your liver and kidneys. We know this is true because even when a person has had his stomach removed surgically so he no longer can absorb vitamin B_{12} it takes a few years before he becomes deficient. A recent report described a vegetarian who was on a B_{12}-deficient diet for twenty-five years before he had any symptoms.

The RDA for vitamin B_{12} is 3 micrograms daily. Most multivitamin preparations contain B_{12} as do some cereals and liquid meals.

* I have been feeling tired lately and a friend suggested that I get B_{12} shots. Will they help?

Many people feel a regular vitamin B_{12} shot makes them "feel great." It may not be helpful but we can assure you it will do no harm. Although B_{12} is essential to every cell in our body, it is rare to have a diet deficient in this nutrient. Even vegetarians who may not eat the liver, meat, eggs, and milk that are good sources of vitamin B_{12} do not become deficient

SOURCES OF VITAMIN B₁₂

Food	Portion	Micrograms of vitamin B₁₂
Milk or yogurt	1 cup	1.0
Egg	1	.6
Cottage cheese	½ cup	.7
Camenbert cheese*	1 ounce	.4
Swiss cheese	1 ounce	.5
Beef liver	3½ ounces	80.0
Tuna fish	3½ ounces	2.2
Ham	3½ ounces	.6
Beef	3½ ounces	1.8
Chicken, broiled	3½ ounces	.4
Crabmeat, canned	3½ ounces	10.0
Flounder	3½ ounces	1.2
Lamb	3½ ounces	2.2
Raw oysters	3½ ounces	18.0
Salmon, canned	3½ ounces	6.9
Veal, lean	3½ ounces	1.8

* As cheese ripens, the amount of B vitamins increases.

easily. A little B_{12} is made by bacteria in the intestine and this, along with what is found in unwashed vegetables and other contaminants (molds, insects, etc.) in foods, seems to be enough. The need for this vitamin is small—only 3 micrograms a day.

Some people become deficient in vitamin B_{12} because they cannot absorb it. This causes a serious condition—pernicious anemia. This form of anemia becomes more common as we age or can happen suddenly after part of the stomach has been removed. These people need B_{12} injections for the rest of their lives.

Some studies have shown that B_{12} shots help relieve "that tired feeling." Critics feel that the lessening of fatigue and sense of well-being reported after the shot is simply due to the placebo effect. In other words, there is the expectation that you will feel better, so you do. Vitamin B_{12} is dark red and that may add to its placebo effect in that it looks like it will "improve" the blood.

In answer to your question, vitamin B_{12} shots will most certainly help a person who has pernicious anemia, but as for others there is little evidence to support the claim that B_{12} is a general tonic. If you wish, you may choose to take a multivitamin supplement rather than the shot. Many supplements contain 5 or 6 micrograms of vitamin B_{12}, an amount greater than your daily need.

Other Vitamins

* Is it true that pantothenic acid can turn my gray hair back to its natural color?

Pantothenic acid is one of a group of vitamins called the "B Complex." In the body it acts as part of a larger molecule that is involved in many metabolic reactions. The name "pantothenic" came from the Greek word *panthos*, which means "everywhere" and that describes where this vitamin can be found—in all foods. In fact, it has been estimated that the average American diet supplies twice as much pantothenic acid as needed. It's not likely that you would be deficient.

Back in 1940, it was found that pantothenic acid could restore the normal black color to rats whose fur had turned gray. A point often overlooked is that the reason the fur turned gray in the first place was because the rats had been fed a synthetic diet lacking pantothenic acid. Loss of hair color due to pantothenic acid deficiency occurs in rats, not in humans. Pantothenic acid in tablets, hair sprays, or in shampoos will not restore color to your hair; in fact the only one who will benefit when you use these products will be the person who sells them to you. Supplements in excess of 10 grams (10,000 mg.) a day may cause diarrhea.

* Will PABA keep my hair from turning gray?

We are sorry to say that we know of no supplement you

can take that will keep your hair from turning gray or turn it back to its former color if it is gray now. (See preceding question.)

PABA (para-aminobenzoic acid), which is part of the B vitamin, folic acid, is useful as a sunscreen. You will see it listed among the ingredients of suntan lotions. The preparations which contain the most are more effective sunscreens.

PABA supplements are sold in 50- and 100-milligram tablets and rather than being beneficial, they are harmful, as they help disease-causing bacteria grow faster and become more resistant to some treatments. Large amounts of PABA, 10 grams or more, can cause a toxic reaction.

* What is vitamin F, and what foods contain it?

There is no vitamin F. You may sometimes see essential fatty acids referred to incorrectly as vitamin F. These essential fatty acids are described more fully in Chapter 8, which deals with high blood pressure and your heart.

Lately we have heard some references to fiber as vitamin F. This is silly because fiber does not fit the definition of a vitamin and will only serve to confuse the consumer.

Other so-called vitamins Q, T, and U that you may have read about in the newspaper have not been shown to be vitamins.

MINERALS

* Is it better to take chelated minerals?

There is no good answer to this question because it would depend on the nature of the chelate and type of mineral. It is not possible to generalize and there has not been enough research done in this area of mineral absorption.

The advertising for chelated minerals that implies better absorption is misleading. It suggests that when minerals, which are inorganic, are bonded (chelated) to protein or other organic substances they are more absorbable. Chelation forms a weak bond and so when the chelated mineral reaches the stomach, the mineral separates from the chelator.

We have been advised by experts that it is a waste of money to pay higher prices for chelated minerals, which may have no value over plain minerals.

MAJOR MINERALS AND THEIR SOURCES

Mineral	*Sources*	*RDA* (*milligrams*)	*U.S. RDA* (*milligrams*)
Calcium	Milk, hard cheese, cottage cheese, leafy green vegetables, shrimp, clams, salmon	800	1,000
Phosphorus	Milk, cheese, eggs, meat, fish, poultry, dried peas and beans, nuts, whole-grain breads and cereals	800	1,000
Magnesium	Whole-grain breads and cereals, dried peas and beans, nuts, milk, meat, green leafy vegetables	300–(females) 350–(males)	400
Sulfur	Eggs, meat, milk, cheese, nuts, dried peas and beans	None given	None given
Sodium	Salt, milk, meat, fish, poultry, eggs, bread	1,100–3,300	None given
Potassium	Meat, fish, poultry, cereals, fruits, vegetables	1,874–5,625	None given
Chlorine	Salt	1,700–5,100	None given

* Will hair analysis tell me what minerals I lack?

Hair analysis is not a reliable way to estimate the amount of minerals in your body. Hair from different places in the body differs greatly in its mineral content and there may be little relationship between the amount of a mineral in the hair and that same mineral in the body.

Hair analysis has been used in research to detect high levels of lead and mercury that would indicate dangerous levels in a population. If you are using a lead acetate hair formula to comb the gray out of your hair, a hair analysis might suggest you are suffering from lead poisoning. Shampoo, hair rinses, tobacco smoke, hard water, and air pollutants can all leave detectable deposits in your hair. Furthermore, it is difficult to get accurate laboratory values because even the testing equipment or laboratory atmosphere can alter results.

Calcium and Phosphorus

* Will calcium supplements prevent periodontal disease?

Almost all of us develop periodontal disease as we get older. It is a disease of the tissue and bone that anchors your teeth into the jaw and is the reason why many of us lose our teeth. (More than 30 percent of Americans aged fifty-five to sixty-four have lost all their teeth.) The exact cause of the disease is not known but it is started by bacterial plaque on the teeth. The disease eventually reaches your jaw bone, causing loss of the minerals the bone is made of.

Anything you can do to reduce dental plaque would reduce your risk of getting severe periodontal disease. Research has shown that cocoa, sharp cheese (like cheddar), and peanuts inhibit the formation of plaque and keep it from sticking to the teeth. It's a good idea to eat these foods at the end of a meal. You may have heard that apples clean your teeth, but they really do not because they are so high in sugar. Don't believe the old saying that an apple is a toothbrush. Raw fibrous foods low in sugar, like celery and carrots, that require a lot of chewing, promote the flow of saliva and that prevents dental plaque.

An adequate diet including optimal fluorine and vitamin D intake, sufficient calcium, and not too much phosphorus, is important in preventing periodontal disease.

Many believe that periodontal disease is a visible sign that bone loss (osteoporosis) is occuring in other parts of the body. Periodontal disease may be followed by osteoporosis in five to ten years. (For more information about osteoporosis see Chapter 5.)

* What foods contain phosphorus?

Americans tend to eat about four times as much phosphorus as they do calcium. It would be better for our bones if we took in about equal amounts of the two minerals. You can help by reducing your intake of phosphorus-rich foods like meat, soda, and processed foods containing phosphorus additives. At the same time, you should increase your intake of calcium so that you get about 1 gram daily. (See the chart "Calcium in Food," Chapter 5.)

Trace Minerals

* What is meant by trace minerals?

The body has fairly large amounts of some minerals like calcium (about 2 pounds in a 120-pound person), phosphorus, magnesium, and sodium (there are others) whose names are familiar to almost everyone. We call these "major minerals," or macrominerals. There is another group of minerals with unfamiliar names. These minerals are in the body in very small amounts. In years past when they did not have the instruments to accurately weigh such small quantities, iron, zinc, copper, manganese, molybdenum, selenium, chromium, iodine, and fluorine, were described as occurring in "traces." These minute amounts can now be accurately measured. The term trace minerals distinguishes those that are required in levels of 50 micrograms to 18 milligrams per day. The copper in one penny could meet our needs for four years. (See the chart "Trace Minerals and Their Sources.")

* How can I be sure that I am getting all the trace minerals I need?

We no longer can give the pat answer that if you eat a balanced diet you are sure to be getting all the trace minerals you need. We now know that many of us get too little of some. It may surprise you to hear that even hospital diets are also deficient.

One way that we can maximize the amount of trace minerals we get is by eating less processed and refined foods (alcohol, soda, sweets). The more whole-grain breads and cereals, whole fruits and vegetables you eat (with peel, when possible, but we don't go so far as to recommend apple cores, as some do), the more likely you are to have enough of the trace minerals.

Trace Minerals* and Their Sources

Mineral	Sources	RDA	U.S. RDA
Chromium	Meat, whole grains	.05–.2 mcg.	None given
Copper	Liver, meat, seafood, whole grains, cocoa, raisins, nuts	2.0–3.0 mg.	2.0 mg.
Fluorine	Fish, tea, wheat germ, meat, spinach, kale, parsley, fluoridated water	1.5–4.0 mg.	None given
Iodine	Seafood, iodized salt	150.0 mcg.	150.0 mcg.
Iron	Organ meat (especially liver), meat, egg yolk, whole wheat, seafood, green leafy vegetables, nuts, dried peas and beans	10.0 mg. (males and females 51+) 18.0 mg. (females under age 50)	18.0 mg.

TRACE MINERALS* AND THEIR SOURCES

Mineral	Sources	RDA	U.S. RDA
Manganese	Bran, soybeans, dried peas and beans, nuts, tea, coffee	2.5–5.0 mg.	None given
Molybdenum	Organ meat, buck-wheat (kasha), meat, whole grains, leafy vegetables, dried peas and beans	.15–.5 mg.	None given
Selenium	Meat, seafood, cereals	.05–.2 mg.	None given
Zinc	Seafood, meat, eggs, whole grains, dried peas and beans	15.0 mg.	15.0 mg.

mg = milligram   mcg = microgram
1,000 mg = 1 g. (1 teaspoon is about 5 grams)
1,000 mcg = 1 mg.

* We have included in this chart only those trace minerals that have an established need in people. Other trace minerals like nickel, silicon, and vanadium are considered essential in animals.

✱ What about supplements for trace minerals? I heard that yeast is good.

Yes, yeast is a good source of some minerals and vitamins too. There really is nothing wrong with taking some yeast, (about one-half of the amount usually recommended on the label) if you like, so long as it does not cause you to have excess gas. (See the question "Is brewer's yeast a good protein supplement?" in Chapter 1).

As for other trace mineral supplements we say "proceed with caution." If you wish to use a multivitamin/mineral preparation that provides the RDA level or less of these minerals, go ahead and take one daily or every other day. That way the amount of the trace mineral in the supplement plus what you get in your food will still fall within a safe range. Remember that toxic levels for many trace minerals may be only a few times greater than what you usually eat.

* How long can I keep minerals before they lose their potency?

You can keep your mineral supplements indefinitely and they will remain potent. Even if they get crumbly or mottled looking they are fine and can be used. This is one instance where the large, economy-size bottle can be used to the very end.

* Will I get enough iodine even though I don't use salt in cooking?

You will probably be getting more than enough iodine even if you don't use a speck of salt!

Iodized salt has been used since the 1930s to prevent iodine deficiency—goiter—in persons who lived far from the coast and so ate a diet low in iodine. The situation is different now. Even though you may be living in an area far from the iodine-containing ocean waters, you are probably eating foods grown in areas where iodine in the soil is plentiful. You are also getting some iodine from unexpected sources. One of these is the air. Iodine is in the air as the result of burning fossil fuels and is absorbed by the body. Sanitizers containing iodine are used in the dairy industry and also for dish washing in restaurants. Some of this iodine finds its way into the food we eat. Some dough conditioners used in bread baking also contain iodine, as do some food colors.

Recent evidence shows that we are getting from four to thirteen times the RDA of iodine. An average liter (35 ounces) of milk contains about 680 micrograms of iodine, this is four times the RDA of iodine (see chart "Trace Minerals and Their Sources"). This means that a single glass of milk daily supplies about all the iodine you need. Rather than worry about not getting sufficient iodine, we are beginning to be concerned with the possibility of getting too much. Don't be concerned about getting an overdose of iodine, as the body normally passes out the excess.

* What foods are the best sources of iron?

Organ meats, especially liver, are best with other sources including meat, egg yolk, whole wheat, seafood, green leafy vegetables, and dried peas and beans. Only a small percentage of the iron in food is absorbed, so that how much is absorbed is as important as the iron content. Until you absorb the nutrient it is really still outside your body even though it is in your intestines. Absorption depends on several factors, one is the type of iron. All of the iron in grains and vegetables is called "nonheme" and it is poorly absorbed compared to "heme" iron. About 40 percent of the total iron in meat, fish, and poultry is heme iron, the remaining 60 percent of the iron is nonheme.

Absorption is affected in other ways as well. When you need iron, your body will absorb more. Eating a vitamin C–rich food (orange, grapefruit, tomato, potato) or some meat, fish, or poultry at a meal will increase the amount of nonheme iron absorbed from all food at that meal. Adding a tomato to a hamburger meal quadruples iron absorption.

Drinking tea with a meal will reduce the quantity of iron you absorb and so will EDTA (ethylenediaminetetraacetic acid)—a food additive, calcium phosphate salts (a calcium supplement), and soy. (See chart "Trace Minerals and Their Sources" for the RDA for iron and see chart "Iron in Foods" for more information.)

* What are enteric-coated iron supplements?

Some people find that iron supplements irritate their stomachs, causing nausea and constipation. Enteric-coated supplements are designed to avoid this as the coating does not dissolve and expose the iron until the tablet is out of the stomach and into the small intestine. This solves the problem

IRON IN FOODS

Food	Portion	Milligrams of iron
Apple	1 medium	0.5
Apricots, dried	4 halves	0.8
Avocado	½	1.3
Bean sprouts	½ cup	0.5
Beef	3 ounces	2.7
Blueberries	⅝ cup	1.0
Bread, white	1 slice	0.6
Bread, whole-wheat	1 slice	0.8
Chickpeas	½ cup	3.0
Corn Muffin	1	0.6
Egg	1	1.1
Chicken, fried	¼	1.8
Grape-nuts	1 ounce	0.5
Green beans	½ cup	0.4
Kidney beans	½ cup	2.2
Liver	3 ounces	8.0
Molasses	1 tablespoon	0.9
Peanuts, roasted	1 tablespoon	0.5
Potato	1 small	0.5
Prunes	4	1.5
Prune juice	½ cup	5.2
Raisins	1 tablespoon	0.4
Split peas, dried	½ cup	1.5
Turkey	3 ounces	1.5
Walnuts	1 tablespoon	0.2

of stomach irritation but reduces the amount of iron absorbed. The iron is released in a place where it is not well absorbed.

If you feel uncomfortable after taking an iron supplement, rather than using enteric-coated tablets, it is better to reduce the number of tablets to one a day. If that is tolerated, gradually add additional tablets, up to the dose required. If this method does not eliminate discomfort, try other types of iron preparations until you find one you can tolerate.

* Will cooking in cast-iron pans help me to get enough iron?

It is true that certain types of food, especially long-cooking acid ones like tomato sauce, will contain more iron if they are cooked in iron pans rather than aluminum, stainless steel, or glass. A study showed that spaghetti sauce cooked in a glass pan contained 3 milligrams of iron in a 3½-ounce portion but when cooked in an iron pan it had over 87 milligrams. In other words, the sauce cooked in an iron pan had twenty-nine times more iron. A similar comparison for scrambled eggs showed that the eggs cooked in an iron pan contained twice as much iron.

Whether or not cooking in iron pots actually will increase your supply of absorbable iron depends on what you cook, your methods of cooking, and how well you care for your cookware. Older, poorly cared for pans give up more iron. If there is rust in the bottom of your pan, don't wipe it out, consider it an iron source.

* My neighbor told me I should be taking selenium. Why do I need it?

Your neighbor may have heard that selenium will prevent cancer. In fact, selenium is both a carcinogen and an anticancer agent. Studies have shown a relation between low selenium intake and the incidence of cancer and also that selenium may prevent cancer, and that some selenium compounds are carcinogens. Obviously much more needs to be known about the cause-and-effect relationship.

Because a low intake of selenium, about 30 micrograms a day, is needed for normal heart function, some people suggest selenium supplements for healthy hearts. However, autopsies found the same levels of selenium in people who died of heart attack or other causes.

It seems that you can get all the selenium you need in food. It's not a good idea to take supplements of trace minerals like selenium without a good reason, because toxic levels may not be more than a few times suggested intakes. (See the chart "Trace Minerals and Their Sources" for more RDA information.)

✳ Will taking a zinc supplement improve my taste buds?

It may, if you are deficient in the mineral. Zinc deficiency causes a loss in taste sensation and this seems to be true even with slight or marginal deficiency. As we all eat fewer calories, more vegetables, and less meat, we may be getting too little zinc.

ZINC* IN FOOD

Food	Portion	Milligrams of zinc
Bagel	1	.53
Banana	1	.30
Beans, dry lima	½ cup	.85
Beans, dry white	½ cup	.95
Beef	3 ounces	3.8
Bologna	1 slice	.50
Bran cereal (40%)	1 ounce	1.0
Bread, white	1 slice	.20
Carrot	1	.30
Cheddar cheese	1 ounce	1.0
Chickpeas	½ cup	1.0
Chicken breast	½	.70
Cottage cheese	½ cup	.52
Egg	1	.5
Farina	½ cup	.10
Lentils	½ cup	1.0
Liver, calf	3 ounces	5.2
Milk	1 cup	.90
Oatmeal	½ cup	.60
Oysters, Atlantic	1 ounce	25.0
Oysters, Pacific	1 ounce	3.0
Peanuts	1 tablespoon	.30
Pineapple juice	½ cup	.19
Spinach	½ cup	.6
Veal	3 ounces	3.6

* The RDA for zinc is 15 mg.

By choosing foods carefully you can meet the RDA for zinc—15 milligrams without a supplement. (See the chart "Zinc in Foods.") If you prefer to have some supplementary zinc, many vitamin-mineral preparations contain zinc. Choose one that does not have more than 15 milligrams. Larger amounts of zinc may interfere with the use of other minerals—copper and calcium. People have been poisoned after eating and drinking foods and beverages stored in galvanized containers because the zinc coating dissolved into the food.

* When I was a little girl I was given arsenic as a tonic because I was underweight. Isn't arsenic a poison?

It is true that arsenic in large amounts is a poison (it has been used as one in lots of detective stories). That does not mean that it cannot be an essential nutrient as well. Many minerals which have essential roles in the body are toxic in amounts just a few times greater than their suggested intakes.

Very small amounts of arsenic have been shown to be needed by animals. In fact, arsenic compounds are sometimes added to poultry and pig feed to stimulate their growth. Human need for arsenic has not been definitely shown but the probability is that it is needed in minute amounts.

Chronic, excessive intake of arsenic either as a tonic or from water supplies or foods has been shown to cause arsenical keratoses, which are precancerous skin lesions. Many adults, like yourself, who took arsenic tonics as children develop these skin lesions. Most adults take in 0.4 to 3.9 milligrams of arsenic daily depending on where they live. Shellfish are rich sources with oysters containing 3 to 10 PPM (parts per million). Saltwater fish average 2 to 8 PPM with fish and shellfish from freshwater having much lower levels.

* Is it safe to cook in aluminum pots?

This question has been debated for forty years or more. Most authorities have felt that so little metal from the aluminum pans dissolved into the food, that there was no problem.

In any case we get much more aluminum from food additives—baking powder and emulsifiers, and from antacids than we get from our pots and pans.

Recently, it has been suggested that aluminum may play a role in some mental disorders. A study of older people showed that those with more aluminum in their bodies were more likely to have poor memory, impaired coordination, and other mental problems. Other studies agree with this.

With this in mind, you might decide to limit your exposure to aluminum in any practical way. For instance, you could cook and store food in glass, porcelain, or stainless steel. (See the question "Will cooking in cast iron pans . . ." in this section.)

3

Other Nutritional Remedies

Do you know that over one-third of the spending power of Americans is in the hands of those forty-five to sixty-four? Over half of their income is discretionary; children are raised, homes furnished, investments matured. They have money to spend and what they want are items that make life comfortable—leisure, entertainment, and travel—in short the "good life."

There is, however, the nagging fear that all this could be lost if their health fails. After all, hasn't Alice recently been complaining about the arthritis pain in her hands; Hank was just told he has high blood pressure; and John, only forty-eight, had a mild heart attack. *You* feel well and want to stay that way.

To postpone, prevent, or minimize the possibility of poor health, many of you over forty have become "health nuts"—jogging, eating health foods, taking vitamins and minerals by the handful, and watching your weight, so that you no longer are preoccupied with getting ill; you are obsessed with staying well.

Advertisers are aware of this preoccupation with good health and use it to make a profit. Health foods, diets, nutrient supplements, and heavily fortified breakfast cereals are all currently being advertised by healthy looking, mature "models." The subliminal message of these ads is that if you use that particular product, read that book, or follow the plan, good health is assured.

You are encouraged to believe that if a little is good a lot must be better, with the result that many of these products are being promoted as far more effective than they actually are. In many cases the nutrient doses suggested are reaching toxic and dangerous levels. "Natural" remedies are suggested for medical disorders, postponing necessary treatment. And even more dangerous is the diet alteration and nutrient self-medication that may be interfering with necessary medication or treatment. People have actually *killed* themselves in the quest for a longer life.

We are not suggesting that all self-treatments, health foods, and nutrient supplements are lethal. Many are helpful, or at the worst harmless. What we are suggesting is that "health" foods do not necessarily promote good health. Some of these *are* safe and reliable and may provide benefits as part of a normal diet; others are unnecessary, costly, and harmful.

Read through the following chapter. You will gain an education in how to protect yourself from nutrition misinformation. As a bonus we will include a few "nutrition" stories you can share with your friends the next time you meet them for lunch or cocktails.

* Are natural foods best?

That's a tough question. We like to rely more heavily on unprocessed foods (fresh fruits and vegetables and whole grains) rather than on highly processed foods (TV dinners, canned soups, and packaged desserts) but the word NATURAL on a food label can often be misleading.

You can snack on Kraft Cracker Barrel Natural Cheddar Cheese sandwiched between Nabisco's Sesame Wheats, "a natural whole-wheat cracker," and wash them both down with Anheuser-Busch Natural Light Beer. But don't stop there—why not feed your dog Gravy Train Dog Food With Natural Beef Flavor, start the day with Quaker 100% Natural Cereals, or enjoy Pillsbury Natural Chocolate Flavored Chocolate Chip Cookies and Wise's Natural Flavor Rippled Potato Chips. Welcome to the world of mass merchandising of "natural" foods.

It is true that many food additives and processing techniques have been questioned and consumers are concerned about the safety of their food supply. However, the word "natural" does not necessarily guarantee that the product is preservative- and additive-free. Natural may be used to modify another word on the product's title. For example, there is a Natural Lemon Flavored Creme Pie available that contains sodium propionate, certified food colors, sodium benzoate, and vegetable gum. The manufacturer claims no deception. The word "natural" was only intended to modify lemon flavor, since the pie contains oil from lemon rinds, a natural flavoring. Even products that have always been preservative- and additive-free, like vinegar, are suddenly being adorned with new NATURAL or NO PRESERVATIVE labels. "Natural" is a current marketing gimmick that is capitalizing on the consumers' desire for good health and their concern about the safety of the food they buy.

To protect the consumer from such marketing strategies, the Federal Trade Commission (FTC), after six years of deliberation, has finally established a legal definition for the term *natural*: "A 'natural' food may not contain artificial or synthetic ingredients and may not be more than 'minimally processed.' Minimal processing includes washing, peeling, canning, bottling or freezing, baking and roasting."

Unfortunately, under this new regulation many foods such as potato chips will be able to qualify as natural as long as the manufacturer fully discloses the ingredients. In this case, natural does not imply good nutrition.

To protect yourself, don't automatically presume that all foods labeled NATURAL are more nutritious than other foods. Be your own best judge of products, look at the ingredients listed, and unit price the item against a similar product not tagged "natural." You may be paying a premium for the word.

* How can you tell when a nutrition claim is fraudulent?

Claims for the miraculous powers of food can be traced back to Eve and the apple. Satan may have been the first nutrition huckster when he disguised himself as a snake!

Today food and nutrition misinformation comes to us disguised as scientific fact. Although the sales pitch may be more sophisticated, the appeal remains the same: the food faddist tries to reach people on an emotional level. For the wrinkled, he promises youth. To those in pain, he promises relief. To a public worried about cancer, he promises a cure. His watchwords are "take control of your own body," "be natural," "live longer," "protect yourself." He subtly or openly attacks doctors, modern technology, and government agencies as part of an ever-growing conspiracy out to get you.

Their business is booming. Americans spend over $1 billion a year on products that promise magical results. No one knows how much of this money is wasted. Frequently there is nothing to substantiate the newly touted claim except anecdotal evidence, testimonials from the famous, or occasionally an antiquated or poorly designed scientific study. Rarely will you find a double-blind study used to prove the product's effectiveness. Double-blind studies are those in which neither the subjects nor investigators know who is receiving the substance to be tested and who is receiving the placebo until after the results are tabulated.

How can you protect yourself? You have started by reading this book. We've presented nutrition facts as we know them—accurately, carefully, and without sensationalism. The message we want you to digest is that moderation and variety in eating are the passwords to good health.

It's not a terribly exciting message but as we, or any other reputable nutritionst will tell you, it is true. Your body is a uniquely complicated machine that functions more efficiently when it is in a state of balance. Too much of a vitamin or mineral, elimination of an entire group of foods (like carbohydrates), or an overabundance of energy (calories) distorts the balance. Moderation and variety are truly the keys to good nutrition. And we can guarantee that good nutrition will enhance the quality of your life.

* Do organically grown foods contain more vitamins and minerals?

Organic enthusiasts seek organic produce to avoid food with chemical and pesticide residues. This makes sense since the question of how much of such chemicals we can safely ingest is still open. They further believe that organic produce is more healthful, than other foods, containing more vitamins and minerals. In fact, there is no scientific proof that organically grown produce is richer in nutrients than plants raised nonorganically. Plants manufacture their own nutrients and absorb others from the soil. If the soil is deficient, it can be compensated for by a chemically manufactured fertilizer or by the release of decomposition products of organic wastes such as animal manure. Natural fertilizers, such as manure, are not problem-free, as we are led to believe. Manure can be high in phosphate and salt, which may damage crops; it may also contain dangerous bacteria, insects, worms, and other pests; and it may even contain toxic chemicals that are the residue from the animal's diet.

As a consumer, the only real benefit you should get from the purchase of organically grown food is the assurance that the products are free of pesticide residue. Unfortunately, tests over the years at various places throughout the country have shown little difference in the level of pesticide residues between organically grown and supermarket produce. In fact, consumers must be wary because more organic produce is *sold* than has been *grown*. Therefore, food is misrepresented as organic.

The problem here is to first define the term "organic foods." There is very little farmland left in the United States that has not at one time been farmed chemically or is not now currently adjacent to such land. If a neighboring farmer sprays pesticides, the wind often carries the spray onto the organic farm. An organic celery farmer in Oregon delivered his crop only to have it judged heavily contaminated with pesticides. Investigation showed that the fields had been flooded at one point in the year and the water brought with it runoff chemicals from nearby farms. Rich Purvis, an owner of an organic farm near San Francisco, concluded that there couldn't be an organic carrot grown in California, even though health food stores there sell them. He explains that soil *must* be chemically treated to destroy nematodes (small worms that attack root crops) and no one has discovered an effective organic way to do it.

Before the consumer can be assured of the quality of organic produce, stricter regulations and testing programs must be established. Currently, Oregon is the only state with a system for defining and testing food to be labeled ORGANI-CALLY GROWN.

* My daughter told me to eat alfalfa as a good source of minerals. Is she right?

Your daughter is mistaken. The claim that alfalfa roots grow deeply into the earth and probe out minerals and trace elements that shallow-rooted plants cannot reach is false. Subsoils are lower in nutrients than topsoils.

One cup of raw alfalfa sprouts contain 23 calories, .8 milligram iron, and 16 milligrams calcium, as well as small amounts of vitamin C and some B vitamins.

A note of caution: if you are an alfalfa sprout lover, eat them in moderation. Alfalfa contains saponins, a naturally occurring food toxicant which, when eaten in large amounts, may damage red blood cells. The saponins in alfalfa increase greatly during sprouting.

* My husband is eating six cloves of raw garlic a day to ward off a heart attack. Is the smell really worth it?

Ancient folklore claims garlic will ward off vampires if worn as an amulet around the neck. Although your husband may be safe from vampires, there is only tentative proof that his practice will prevent a heart attack.

Recent research data has suggested that when large quantities of raw garlic are eaten regularly there may be a lowering of serum cholesterol, triglyceride levels, and low-density lipoprotein (LDL), while at the same time increasing high-density lipoproteins (HDL). This result occurred in healthy people as well as those who have coronary heart disease. Two drawbacks to this discovery are: garlic has to be eaten for a long period of time—eight months or longer—and a person has to eat 30 grams of raw garlic each day (this is equivalent to twenty peeled, medium garlic cloves).

Further, garlic kills certain types of bacteria and there have been claims that it is more effective than usual antibiotics. Garlic power and garlic pills do not have the same action.

The smell you are experiencing occurs when garlic is eaten in large amounts. The substances that are in garlic and onions that cause "bad breath" are absorbed into the bloodstream and exhaled from the lungs. Because of this, no amount of mouthwash can remove the odor.

* Can lecithin, taken daily, reduce a high blood cholesterol?

Lecithin is a *phospholipid*, a type of fat that makes up a small portion of the fat you eat. In food processing, lecithin is used as an *emulsifier*, a substance that keeps fat evenly dispersed, as in a salad dressing that never separates. Lecithin is found in egg yolk, milk, soybeans, and corn. It is sold in capsules, liquid, and granules, and is a popular supplement.

Because of its emulsifying properties, it has been claimed that lecithin supplements can reduce high serum cholesterol and dissolve fatty deposits in blood vessels. These claims are untrue. The lecithin you eat in food or take in capsule or granule form does not reach your blood vessels intact. The enzymes lecithinase, found in your intestines, breaks down lecithin before it passes through the intestinal wall. The lecithin your body needs for normal functioning, such as building cell membranes and aiding in the transport of fat, is made from scratch by the liver from the by-products of digestion. Dietary supplements of additional lecithin are not necessary. (See the question "I seem to be getting increasingly absent-minded . . ." in this chapter for more information on lecithin.) Right now, researchers are exploring the value of daily lecithin supplements, and in the future we may have more information to share.

Further, claims have been made that lecithin can eliminate liver spots, relieve arthritic pain, help dry skin and psoriasis, and improve memory. Sorry—these claims are unsubstantiated as well.

* What Chinese food clears clogged arteries?

Dr. Dale E. Hammerschmidt of the University of Minnesota recently reported that tree ears, an edible Chinese fungus, possesses anticlotting properties that may account for the low incidence of coronary artery disease in China.

The fungus, also called "black tree fungus," "cloud ear," "wood ears," or "mo-er" is a common ingredient in many traditional Chinese dishes. In fact, the Chinese regard mo-er as a longevity tonic.

Biochemists at George Washington University have identified the anticlotting substance in the fungus as adenosine, a chemical also present in garlic and onion. Adenosine interfers with the clumping of blood cells, called "platelets," which play a crucial role in blood clot formation. This food may someday prove to be an effective tool in the prevention of atherosclerosis.

* What is the nutrient that works like a sleeping pill?

Recent evidence indicates that there is a relationship between our diet and our brain function. The ability of the brain to make and release three of the fifteen known neurotransmitters—serotonin, acetylcholine, and norepinephrine—depends on the nutrient content of the last meal eaten. The ability to transmit impulses between nerve cells is dependent on the chemical neurotransmitters.

Tryptophan, an amino acid, found in high amounts in animal proteins, is the precursor of the neurotransmitter serotonin. When you eat a meal high in carbohydrate, which contains no animal protein, there is an elevation of brain tryptophan and stimulation of serotonin synthesis.

In controlled experiments, subjects who reported they were unable to sleep were treated successfully by giving them 5 to 10 grams of tryptophan. This level of tryptophan supplementation far exceeds that which would be obtained from food and far exceeds the normal nutritional needs of the body. Therefore, self-medication with tryptophan supplements for sleep disturbances should be approached with caution. (See the following two questions for more information on neurotransmitters.)

* I seem to be getting increasingly absentminded. Can any nutrient stimulate the mind?

In the brain, memory seems to depend on the level of the neurotransmitter acetylcholine. Choline is the precursor of acetylcholine. It can either be made in the body or eaten in foods such as egg yolks, dried beans, and wheat germ.

Choline supplements, to increase the brain level of acetylcholine, have been used to treat Alzheimer's disease, which is believed to be the most common form of dementia in people over age forty-five. Choline supplements slowed the progress of this condition when given in the disease's early stages. Researchers hope to prove that additional choline may help to improve our memory as we age.

Lecithin, a choline-containing compound, is often suggested as a memory-stimulating substance. Commercial lecithin may in fact contain little choline.

* Are there mood-elevating foods, and how much should you eat?

The neurotransmitter norephinephrine is produced by the brain from the amino acid tyrosine. Besides its many other functions in the body, norepinephrine is involved in mood regulation. It has been speculated that manipulation of tyrosine levels in the brain may prove useful in treating mood disorders such as depression. Not enough research has been done to recommend supplementation with tryosine, but some day it may be possible to successfully treat psychiatric disorders through diet changes.

* Can herbs be used safely in place of medicine?

Folklore would have us believe that yarrow cures baldness, agrimony cures forgetfulness, hemlock cures lust (permanently), angelica cures deafness, dill combats witchcraft, and fennel increases the life-span.

On the serious side, many of our modern medicines had their origins in plants—foxglove yields digitalis, poppies are made into morphine, and aloe vera soothes burns.

Some common herbal remedies seem to be safe and may be effective. Garlic chewed or brewed into a tea is recommended for upper respiratory infections. Under laboratory conditions, garlic does inhibit bacterial growth.

Cinnamon tea and regular tea helps stop simple diarrhea. The tannins in the teas appear to be the effective ingredient. Many of the illnesses with suggested herbal remedies are self-limiting, therefore the illness will disappear in a short while whether treated or not. (Colds or diarrhea will normally go away in a few days.)

Although herbs are natural they still may contain potent chemicals in unknown quantities. Often people are buying and using herbs with little understanding of their possible side effects. Cases have been reported of reactions that range from mild diarrhea to violent hallucinations.

If you are considering herbal remedies we suggest you observe the following precautions.

1. Check with a pharmacist about safety.
2. Use only small amounts.
3. Don't mix herbal remedies with other medicines.
4. Don't harvest your own herbs.
5. If you are ill, seek a doctor's advice even if you plan to try an herbal remedy.
6. Remember, herbal preparations should be classified as drugs not foods.

(See the following question for more information on herbal remedies.)

* I enjoy herbal teas but have been warned they can cause bad reactions. Is this true?

A forty-three-year-old woman drank a cup of tea made of powdered poke-root purchased at a health food store. Within thirty minutes she experienced nausea and vomiting, cramps, and abdominal pain, which lead to watery and then bloody diarrhea. Rushed to the hospital, she was experiencing irregular heart rhythms and very low blood pressure. It took twenty-four hours to stabilize her condition.

An older couple, hoping for relief from arthritis, died after drinking tea prepared from the leaves of foxglove.

A woman who drank tea made from two ground nutmegs was treated for a rapid pulse, incoherent speech, and hallucinations. She believed monsters were attempting to devour her.

In our quest for health and desire to limit caffeine, herbal teas have enjoyed a resurgence of popularity. Many herbal teas do not and are not required to list ingredients, additionally the herbs vary in potency and herbal tea mixtures vary from batch to batch. You can see why a person may have a bad reaction.

Following is a brief list of some of the reactions we've come across:

Diarrhea—buckthorn bark, senna, dock root, aloe leaves

Nervous system disruptions—catnip, juniper, hydrangea, lobelia, jimsonweed, wormwood, burdock, nutmeg

Allergic reactions—chamomile, goldenrod, marigold, yarrow

Increased sun sensitivity—Saint-John's-wort

Cardiovascular toxicity—licorice, foxglove

Poisons—Indian tobacco, mistletoe, pokeweed, inkberry

Carcinogens—sassafras (banned for sale in U.S. by FDA)

We would recommend that you use only those herbal teas that disclose all their ingredients on the label. Don't be a purist and harvest your own ingredients by the roadside. And if you should ever experience any unusual reactions, contact your doctor immediately.

✴ I think I need a daily pick-me-up. Would a ginseng tonic be useful?

Ginseng has been used by man for thousands of years as a health tonic, stimulant, and aphrodisiac. One of the most popular herbs in use, it can be purchased in liquid, powder, or capsule form and is often brewed into tea. One teamaker advertised his ginseng tea to ". . . guarantee joyful temper, plenty of pure red blood and relief from your irritable bladder." In the United States alone, it is estimated that there are 5 to 6 million ginseng users.

Ginseng is classified, pharmacologically, as an adaptogen because experimental studies suggest that it may help the body adapt to stress and correct adrenal and thyroid dysfunction. Because of the stress-relief concept, ginseng consumption is often suggested during menopause. Research in the United States, in this area, is inconclusive, but many internationally reputable scientists are looking more closely at the properties of the ginseng plant.

Occasional use of a ginseng preparation would probably cause little or no harm and may be helpful to the user. Appropriate daily doses of ginseng are impossible to estimate since it is sold in so many forms. Many products, like the teas and tonics, contain 88 to 95 percent milk sugar and only a dash of ginseng. Doses as low as 0.5 gram have been reported to be therapeutically effective. Only you can determine whether a ginseng tonic would be the daily "pick-me-up" you feel you need.

One thing we can tell you, if you choose to use a ginseng product daily, use it in low moderate doses. Dr. Ronald Seigel of the University of California has recently identified a Ginseng Abuse Syndrome (GAS). A number of ginseng users that Dr. Seigel studied suffered from common symptoms— hypertension together with nervousness, sleeplessness, skin eruptions, morning diarrhea. He concluded that long-term consumption of large amounts of ginseng (3 grams or more daily) is associated with hypertension and stimulation of the central nervous system. So remember, a little may be helpful but a lot can be harmful and possibly even dangerous.

* Can yogurt smooth wrinkles?

Yogurt is one of the few current fad foods that can boast of respectability. It will not help you to live past one-hundred or lower blood cholesterol, but it may be better digested by those intolerant to milk, and it is a good source of calcium.

Yogurt has a long history of curative powers. The Turks

believed it cured insomnia, Persian women used it to banish wrinkles, and Dr. John Harvey Kellogg (of cereal fame) used it to cleanse the bowel. Today doctors are recommending yogurt for patients on antibiotics, in the belief that the live organisms in the yogurt will help replace the body's friendly intestinal bacteria killed by the antibiotics. We now know that acidophilus milk is more effective than yogurt in replacing intestinal bacteria.

Yogurt is a good food with all the nutrients found in the milk from which it was made, but it can offer no magical promises of good health or longevity.

* A friend of mine told me she is douching with yogurt. Why would that be beneficial?

In some women vaginal yeast and monilial infections (caused by the fungi Candida) are quite bothersome. In menopausal women the incidence of these infections is higher due to lower estrogen levels, vaginal dryness, and the greater number of vaginal operations this age group has. Douching with plain yogurt containing lactobacillus acidophilous cultures (these are the most common cultures found in yogurt) appears to control the growth of the infectious organisms in the vagina.

If your friend is troubled with recurrent vaginal infections the yogurt douche may prove helpful. Also helpful is wearing cotton underpants and not wearing pantyhose or slacks. Of course it goes without saying that your friend should be visiting her doctor regularly.

* Does wheat germ contain an antiaging factor?

Claims that wheat germ can prolong life come from a book called *Everything You Always Wanted to Know About Wheat Germ*, where the author states in the preface that wheat germ helps ". . . create cellular-tissue rejuvenation in the body and mind." It has also been claimed that wheat germ can cure heart disease, improve fertility, and increase virility. Go ahead and sprinkle wheat germ on yogurt, cereal, or other foods—but do so for its crunchy nutlike flavor, not for its curative properties.

Wheat germ contains B vitamins, vitamin E, and protein. It can be a nutritious addition to a varied diet, but keep in mind that 1 ounce (three tablespoons) contains 102 Calories.

* What is rutin which my friend takes for her arthritis?

Rutin is a member of the group of substances called "bioflavonoids." They are found naturally in red peppers and in the juice and peel of citrus fruits. You may find bioflavonoids sold in stores as "vitamin P," even though the American Chemical Society disqualified them as a vitamin in the early 1950s. A deficiency of bioflavonoids has never been demonstrated in man or animals.

The success of rutin, hesperidin (another bioflavonoid), or vitamin P comes from its emotional appeal. People are induced to believe in a magical cure and made to feel uneasy if they do not heed the warnings. Some unproven "cures" attributed to bioflavonoids are relief from rheumatoid arthritis, arteriosclerosis, hypertension, and the common cold.

Rutin is often sold in capsule form in combination with vitamin C. This combination has recently been reported as beneficial in treating fever blisters or cold sores. If you or someone you know is bothered by these recurrent sores, take 200 milligrams of bioflavonoids plus 200 milligrams of vitamin C three times daily for three days, when you feel the fever blisters forming. In many cases the blisters will either not erupt, or, if they do, you will have them for a shorter period of time.

* Will apple cider vinegar help the arthritis pain in my hand?

In the late 1950s Dr. DeForest Jarvis recommended apple cider vinegar as a cure for arthritis in his book *Folk Medicine: A Vermont Doctor's Guide to Good Health.* He claimed the acid in vinegar would remove calcium deposits in arthritic joints. Jarvis proposed his theory after watching plumbers remove calcium deposits on pipes by the use of an acid solution. For years, the medical community refuted Jarvis's claim, stating repeatedly that methods used to treat household plumbing can not be extrapolated into medical treatment for the arthritis sufferer. Efforts of the medical and scientific community were of no avail since Jarvis published a sequel, *Arthritis and Folk Medicine*, which is still selling today.

We doubt seriously that you will find any relief from your arthritis pain if you take apple cider vinegar. No food will cause arthritis nor will any food cure it. Arthritis is a chronic condition, and as with any chronic condition, a balanced diet and a state of good nutritional health will serve as a positive aid to the treatment prescribed. (See Chapter 9 for more information on arthritis.)

✱ Can blackstrap molasses help varicose veins?

Claims that blackstrap molasses can cure ulcers, varicose veins, and arthritis, prevent cancer, induce sleep, correct nervousness, or restore gray hair to its natural color should be disregarded. There have been no verified cases to support these claims.

Blackstrap molasses is the thick, syrupy residue left behind after sugar refining is complete. It is a simple product, used mostly in rural areas until Gayelord Hauser became its champion in his 1951 book *Look Younger, Live Longer*. Hauser claimed blackstrap molasses to be a "wonder" food because it was rich in B vitamins, calcium, and iron. One tablespoon does contain 116 milligrams calcium and 2.3 milligrams iron along with 43 Calories. As for Hauser's claim that blackstrap molasses is "rich" in B vitamins, you would need to eat between forty and seventy-five tablespoons to meet your daily need for the B vitamins riboflavin, niacin, and thiamine.

4

What You Should Know About Caffeine, Alcohol, and Drugs

[The] desire to take medicine is perhaps the greatest
feature which distinguishes man from animals.
—Sir William Osler (1849–1919), physician

Have you had a cup of coffee today? A drink? Taken any medication? Most of these seem relatively harmless, but are you aware each interacts with your nutrition and may interact with each other resulting in dangerous side effects. We're not suggesting you stop drinking coffee, become a teetotaler, and start seeing a faith healer—but we are going to raise questions about some commonplace practices that should be given further thought.

Caffeine

The first coffee was eaten, not sipped, by African tribes who crushed wild coffee berries, mixed them with fat, and ate the coffee balls in war parties. Far from the social cup of coffee we know today! Coffee has traveled the world, arriving in the United States after patriots dumped 342 cases of tea into Boston Harbor in 1773. Prior to this, coffee was not a popular drink in the Colonies but it was used. Even the *Mayflower*'s cargo included a mortar and pestle for grinding coffee beans. Today the U.S. is the world's largest coffee importer but coffee consumption is down. Why? Because people have become suspicious of caffeine. Even the Federal Drug Administration has removed it from the GRAS (Generally Recognized As Safe) list and is regulating it as an interim food additive until further studies are completed.

Is all the concern warranted? Are all the accusations against caffeine true? Yes and no. Concern is healthy and we should continuously question the safety of foods we eat, but we also need to sort out the sensational from the factual. We'll do that for you, starting by giving you a "safe" amount of coffee or tea to drink each day, showing you hidden sources of caffeine, such as Anacin and orange soda, discussing the "charges" against caffeine, and coming to a verdict. In some cases, caffeine is guilty and should be removed from the diet. But in other cases—such as heart disease and cancer—the evidence seems circumstantial.

Alcohol

A fifty-six-year-old businessman, just diagnosed as a diabetic and beginning to use Orinase, an antidiabetic drug, goes to a business lunch and orders a cocktail. Within minutes after finishing the drink he experiences flushing, a rapid heartbeat, and clutches his chest. His luncheon companion has him rushed to the hospital, presumably with a heart attack, actually it is an alcohol-drug reaction.

Alcohol does not mix well with antibiotics, anticoagulants, antidiabetic drugs, antihistamines, high blood pressure drugs, antidepressants, and sedatives. At the same time, alcohol is part of over five-hundred oral medications. Alcohol-drug interactions can be serious and often occur because you are unaware of the consequences of this combination. You know not to mix drinking and narcotics such as codeine, or with tranquilizers like Valium, but are you aware that alcohol can react with Alka-Seltzer, Bufferin, Tylenol, and Dristan?

On a more positive note, we can prescribe a drink a day as a potential life extender. Alcohol is like a two-faced coin—it has a negative as well as positive side. We'll tell you about both. We even know how to work a drink into a diabetic or low-sodium diet. Weight watchers can have one, too.

Drugs

What do drugs have to do with nutrition? By the time you finish this chapter, you'll never ask that question again. Drugs can block the use of vitamins and minerals in the body and vitamins and minerals can inactivate drugs. Take a drug when your stomach is full and it may never be absorbed and used. Take other drugs on an empty stomach and you may cause irritation and bleeding. Is it a full stomach or an empty one? We've sorted that out with two handy charts, "Drugs to Take on an Empty Stomach" and "Drugs to Take with Meals."

Most commonly, foods and beverages interfere with absorption of drugs. A classic example is the one with tetracycline antibiotics and dairy foods in which the calcium in milk, cheese, and yogurt prevents absorption almost completely. On the other hand, taking iron supplements with citrus fruits or juices increases our normal absorption rate of the iron. Some drugs interfere with our use of nutrients leading to nutrient depletion. As little as 2½ tablespoons of mineral oil a day can reduce the body's use of vitamins A, D, and K. Long-term use of diuretics, "water pills," can lead to serious potassium depletion. Of the eight top selling drugs in 1980 *all* of them had a nutritional side effect. See the table "Top Selling Drugs in U.S." on the following page. Do you see any medication you regularly take?

Caffeine, alcohol, and drugs are all perfectly legal substances with potentially hazardous effects when improperly used. Read through the remainder of the chapter so you'll know how to use all three to your advantage and well-being.

CAFFEINE

* Should I stop drinking coffee?

That's a question we can't answer with a decided yes or no. In certain situations reducing or eliminating coffee can be beneficial. Women with benign breast disease have found marked relief from cyclic pain when coffee and other foods

TOP-SELLING DRUGS IN U.S.*

Drug	Disease or function	Reaction that may interfere with normal food intake
Tagamet	peptic ulcer	malabsorption of nutrients, diarrhea, constipation
Valium	muscle relaxant, tranquilizer	stimulates appetite
Inderal	heart disease, hypertension, migraine headache	dry mouth, constipation, nausea, vomiting, diarrhea, decreased carbohydrate tolerance
Motrin	arthritis	reacts with alcohol; nausea, stomach pains, heartburn, bloating, gas, vomiting, diarrhea, constipation, water retention, reduced appetite
Aldomet	hypertension	reacts with alcohol; need additional vitamin B_{12} and folic acid; weight gain, water retension, diarrhea, nausea, vomiting, gas, sore tongue, constipation
Dyazide	hypertension	reacts with alcohol; dry mouth, nausea, vomiting, diarrhea, affects nutrient levels in the body
Keflex	antibiotic	sore mouth, diarrhea, nausea, stomach cramps; may give a false-positive result for sugar in the urine
Clinoril	arthritis	gastrointestinal pains, impaired digestion, nausea, diarrhea, gas, constipation, lack of appetite, water retention, weight gain, inflammation of the stomach

*Listed in descending order of sales, based on 1980 figures from Oppenheimer and Company.

were removed from their diet. (See Chapter 5 for more complete information.) People with recurrent anxiety attacks may not realize that they are experiencing a caffeine overdose with reactions that include dizziness, agitation, restlessness, recurring headaches, and sleep difficulties. Those who drank eight to fifteen cups of coffee a day reported these "anxiety-like" attacks. At times, the attacks became so disturbing that a doctor was consulted and tranquilizers were prescribed. Long standing and unresolved allergies, migraine headaches, chronic vomiting, and vaginal ulcers have all been relieved when coffee or tea were avoided. In many of these cases the intake was excessive—twenty cups of coffee a day. Most of us do not habitually drink this amount. But what about the five, seven, or ten cups we do drink each day. Should we?

Our advice would be to go easy. Three cups of coffee or four cups of tea is an amount that is conservatively safe and seems to cause no disturbing symptoms. Read the remaining questions on caffeine in beverages and drugs. Calculate your average daily consumption. Now you decide—"Should I stop drinking coffee?"

* What exactly is caffeine?

Caffeine is a stimulant found in coffee, tea, carbonated beverages, cocoa, chocolate, and medications. Although not addictive, it is habit forming and the body comes to depend on its use. The average daily caffeine intake in the United States is approximately 206 milligrams, or the equivalent of two-and-one-quarter cups of coffee. We get most of our caffeine in coffee, tea, or soda; only tiny amounts are taken in through chocolate beverages and foods. Some people, however, take significant amounts in over-the-counter caffeine-containing drugs. (See the table on page 85.)

Caffeine is rapidly absorbed from the digestive tract, entering tissue and organs within minutes. A "lift" can be experienced within a half-hour and continue for three and one-half hours. The maximum effect on the central nervous system is felt in one hour, stimulating the cortex and the heart muscle, increasing the urge to urinate, and improving the capacity for mental and physical work. The "stay awake" or "pick-me-up" properties have been clearly shown. Doses

SOURCES OF CAFFEINE

Beverages	Milligrams of caffeine (per 5 ounces)
Coffee	
percolated	110–125*
drip	146–181*
instant	53–100*
decaffeinated	2–4*
Pero (instant cereal beverage)	0
Postum	0
Tea	
black	50†
green	30†
instant hot tea	45
canned ice tea	9–15‡
instant ice tea	60
regular ice tea	56‡
Hot cocoa	5
Cocoa-sugar mix (water added)	5

Chocolate	(per 1 ounce)
Milk chocolate candy	6
Chocolate candy	23
Baking chocolate	45
Carob	0

* Depends on strength of the brew.

† Caffeine content will increase with length of steeping time.

‡ In both cases, figures are based on a 5-ounce serving of tea; however, canned ice tea comes in a 12-ounce can, increasing caffeine content from 22 to 36 milligrams; ice tea figures are based on 11.5 milligrams caffeine per fluid ounce.

of 150 to 300 milligrams (the equivalent of two to two and one-half cups of coffee) eliminate fatigue and boredom, and increase accuracy in physical and mental tasks for a short time.

Man has sought the effect of caffeine for centuries. Stone Age man discovered and brewed beverages from caffeine-containing plants, the Chinese drank tea in the eighth century, and Arabians brewed coffee in the ninth century. Today every human society has a caffeine-containing food or

CAFFEINE CONTENT OF DRUGS

Prescription medication	Milligrams of caffeine (per tablet)
APCs (aspirin, phenacetin, and caffeine)	32
Cafergot	100
Darvon Compound	32
Norgesic	30

Nonprescription medication	Milligrams of caffeine (per tablet)
Anacin	32
Aqua-Ban	200
Bromoquinine	15
Bromo-Seltzer	32
Cope	32
Coricidin	30
Coryban-D	30
Dexatrim	200
Dietac	200
Dristan	30
Excedrin	60
Midol	32
No-Doz	100
Pre-Mens Forte	100
Prolamine	280
Sinarest	30
Triaminican	30
Vivarin	200

beverage as a staple in its diet: the English and others use tea; Arabia, Indonesia, Brazil, and the United States rely on coffee; South American countries use cocoa beverages; and many exotic foods, drinks, and gums are found in other areas around the globe. Worldwide, caffeine-containing beverages have evolved into popular, acceptable drinks.

* Is caffeine dangerous?

Caffeine was first isolated from coffee beans in 1820. It is odorless with a bitter taste and very soluble in hot water. In spite of over 150 years of scientific studies there is still much to learn about this popular stimulant.

Caffeine is one of the few common foods that acts as a drug in the body in the amounts we usually consume. Two hundred milligrams of caffeine is considered a pharmacologically active dose, a level easily achieved by drinking less than two cups of coffee. Regular caffeine consumption in excess of four cups of coffee a day can lead to a dependence on caffeine with definite bodily discomfort when caffeine is withdrawn or reduced.

What are the dangers in consuming this stimulant regularly? Some of the adverse effects of caffeine have been known for a long time—sleep disturbances; mood changes such as anxiety, depression, and irritability; heartburn and stomach upsets. Currently, caffeine is being reexamined for other potential harmful effects.

It has been suggested that caffeine may cause birth defects and contribute to heart disease, hypertension, bladder cancer, peptic ulcer, and cystic breast disease. Although in all these areas the research is incomplete, in the next few questions we'll examine the facts as we know them. But before we go on, an important note must be made with regard to cigarette smoking.

Smoking is a significant risk factor for birth defects, heart disease, hypertension, peptic ulcers, and cystic breast disease. Further, we know that cigarette smokers drink more coffee than nonsmokers. Why? Smokers clear caffeine from their bodies as much as 55 percent faster than do nonsmokers. It is speculated that smokers would drink more coffee to sustain the desired "lift" from caffeine. Therefore, it is often difficult to appropriately assess caffeine as a risk factor since many who report high caffeine intakes also smoke. Which poses the risk—cigarettes, caffeine, or the combination of the two?

* Does caffeine cause cancer?

Coffee drinking has been linked to cancer of the liver, bladder, kidney, and pancreas. The research used to support these claims was often anecdotal or fraught with inaccuracies so that is was difficult to duplicate and validate. Therefore, the carcinogenicity of caffeine remains controversial.

Coffee is a complex chemical compound, containing more than three hundred substances of which caffeine is but one. Caffeine is not the only substance in coffee that has been linked to bladder cancer. Tar and other chemicals formed when coffee is roasted have caused bladder cancer in guinea pigs even when no caffeine was present. Researchers at the Harvard School of Public Health recently reported evidence that drinking two cups of coffee a day may double the risk of cancer of the pancreas. The news was alarming and made headlines nationwide. What made less sensational news was the fact the authors of the research said their results were preliminary and suggestive only of further study. The Harvard study also showed that pancreatic cancer risk was not elevated in tea drinkers, a beverage with substantial amounts of caffeine. If, in the future, coffee consumption and the incidence of pancreatic cancer are linked, chances are it will be due to another substance than caffeine found in coffee. These examples clearly show that definite evidence linking caffeine and the risk of cancer is still elusive and much more research is needed before an association can be made.

To explore the flip side of this issue, there is some evidence caffeine may be anticarcinogenic and actually helpful in treating cancer. When caffeine is given in combination with radiation therapy or anticancer drugs, the effectiveness of these treatments seems to increase. Caffeine appears to prevent cancer cells from repairing themselves, hence making them more liable to destruction by radiation and drugs and less likely to spread quickly. But don't jump the gun—caffeine is not a cancer cure. More research and work needs to be done in this area as well.

For more information see the question in Chapter 9 "Are coffee enemas useful in treating cancer?" and the question "Will drinking decaffeinated coffee increase my chances of getting cancer?" in this section.

* How can I reduce my caffeine intake?

When you have read through the following questions, you'll be aware of which foods contain caffeine, so obviously these are the ones to limit or eliminate. It is wise, however, not to abruptly remove all these foods at once, particularly if you are a heavy caffeine consumer.

People who habitually drink tea, coffee, or cola throughout the day may find they suffer "caffeine withdrawal" when they suddenly stop these drinks. The symptoms occur twelve to sixteen hours after the last caffeine dose—headache, irritability, nausea, vomiting, mental depression, drowsiness, and disinterest in work. The discomfort can last up to seventy-two hours. To minimize "withdrawal," heavy caffeine consumers should gradually wean themselves off caffeine over a period of a few days to a week. If you drink ten cups of coffee a day, cut down to eight at first, don't accept refills, and look for alternative beverages at and between meals. After a few days, cut down to six, then four, until you are no longer drinking any coffee. You may replace some of your coffee with decaffeinated or noncoffee substitutes, like Postum or Pero, to retain the pleasure of a hot beverage. Some people find they can drink a limited amount of coffee, such as a "morning cup," and substitute other beverages during the rest of the day.

Only you can decide how much caffeine is too much for you, but remember we've suggestd an upper limit of three cups of coffee or four cups of tea a day as a reasonable amount.

✳ How much caffeine is in a cup of coffee?

Coffee remains our largest source of caffeine with an average yearly consumption of twenty-eight gallons. The caffeine from this amount of coffee will vary depending on how the coffee is brewed. Automatic drip coffeepots brew the strongest cupful of caffeine. Instant coffee gives us the least. Brewing time is also important. The longer the coffee grounds and the water are in contact the more caffeine will be extracted. Extended perking or reperking coffee increases its caffeine content and gives it a bitter flavor. (See the chart "Sources of Caffeine.")

Note: Reheating coffee does not affect its caffeine content.

✳ Which has more caffeine, coffee or tea?

Black and oolong teas have more caffeine per pound than coffee. A pound of tea, however, makes 240 cups while a pound of ground coffee makes 50 to 60 cups, resulting in less caffeine per cup of tea.

The length of steeping time effects the caffeine content.

One-minute brew	9–33 milligrams
Three-minute brew	20–46 milligrams
Five-minute brew	20–50 milligrams

To minimize your caffeine intake, allow your tea leaves or teabag to steep one minute or less, or try drinking green tea, which is lower in caffeine. (See the chart "Sources of Caffeine" for more information on the caffeine content of tea.)

✳ Which brand of tea has the least caffeine?

This is a difficult question, since there are so many variables: bagged versus loose versus instant preparations; differences in brewing methods; and personal preference for strength. Imported teas, generally, have more caffeine than domestic brands. Of the domestic brands, regardless of strength of brew, Red Rose contained the most caffeine followed by Salada, Lipton, and Tetley.

* Someone told me there is caffeine in soda. Is that true?

Most of the caffeine extracted from coffee—about 2 million pounds per year—is purchased by beverage manufacturers and added to soda pop. Approximately 10 percent of the caffeine consumed each year is in soda.

Is the use of caffeine as a food additive safe? Manufacturers report using caffeine as a flavor enhancer, a flavoring agent, and a synergist. Kola nut extract, which naturally contains caffeine, provides about 10 percent of the caffeine normally found in cola drinks. The remaining 90 percent is added. It is the added caffeine that is currently being questioned by the FDA.

Until caffeine as a food additive is conclusively proven safe, the FDA has removed it from the GRAS (Generally Recognized As Safe) list and is regulating it as an interim food additive. Interim status recognizes that a substance is under question but allows the substance continued use until these questions are answered by further study. This interim status is only granted when there is reasonable certainty that no public harm will result. The FDA is requiring studies to resolve questions concerning the possibility of caffeine as a risk in birth defects, behavior disturbances, and cancer. While the studies are being done, all foods with added caffeine will be required to state CAFFEINE on the ingredient label. This will allow consumers to identify caffeine-containing foods and limit their exposure.

See the chart "Caffeine Content of Carbonated Beverages." You would expect to find Coke, Pepsi, and other cola-type beverages listed, but did you realize citrus-flavored soda—Mountain Dew, Mellow Yellow, and Sunkist Orange—are also high in caffeine? Among the ten best-selling soft drinks, only two—7-Up and Sprite—contain no added caffeine.

Caffeine Content of Carbonated Beverages

Carbonated beverages	Milligrams of caffeine (per 12-ounces)
Mountain Dew	54
Mellow Yellow	51
Shasta Cola	42
Dr Pepper	38
Sugar Free Dr Pepper	38
Pepsi Cola	38
Royal Crown (RC) Cola	37
Diet Royal Crown (RC) Cola	37
Diet Rite Cola	34
Diet Pepsi	34
Coca-Cola	33
Mr. Pibb	33
Tab	32
7-Up	0
Sprite	0
RC-100 (Royal Crown)	0
Patio Orange	0
Fresca	0
Hires Root Beer	0
Pepsi Free	0
Pepsi Free (Diet)	0

* Are the new "cereal-filled" coffee products better to drink than regular coffee?

Chicory root, from the endive plant, has been used as a coffee extender for centuries. Popular in the South, it is currently undergoing a revival as people wish to cut their caffeine intake. Chicory may be brewed by itself but is more likely to be mixed with ground coffee—1½ tablespoons ground chicory to 3 tablespoons ground coffee.

General Foods is marketing Mellow Roast, a mixture of coffee, bran, wheat, and molasses with 42 milligrams caffeine per cup. A new reduced-caffeine coffee, Lite, is marketed by McLaughlin's Manor House. This coffee has one-third less caffeine per cup.

If you want to limit caffeine and do not wish to use decaffeinated coffee, these products may be the answer.

* Are there vitamins in coffee?

The nutritional value of coffee is limited; however a cup of coffee does provide 5 Calories, 5 milligrams calcium, 5 milligrams phosphorus, .2 milligram of iron, 10 micrograms thiamine, 10 micrograms riboflavin, and .9 milligram niacin. Based on an adult's daily nutrient need, all of these amounts are negligible except for niacin. Three cups of coffee a day would provide approximately 18 percent of the daily niacin need of men and 25 percent for women.

One cup of tea provides 2 Calories, 5 milligrams calcium, 4 milligrams phosphorus, 2 milligrams iron, .1 to .2 milligram fluoride, 40 micrograms riboflavin, .1 milligram niacin, and 1 milligram vitamin C. Even if four cups were drunk everyday, the level of nutrients found in tea is so low it would not add significantly to the daily need for any nutrient except fluoride.

* Can coffee drinking increase my risk of heart disease?

Finally we can give you a definite answer! Coffee drinking will not increase your risk of heart disease nor will it increase serum cholesterol. Numerous carefully controlled scientific studies have found no evidence that coffee, in moderation, will increase the risk of heart disease. Coffee as a cause of strokes has also been ruled out. Some doctors, however, still continue to limit coffee and caffeine intake in cardiac patients. If these foods are used with moderation, there is no reason to restrict them.

Note: If a person suffers from heart rhythm abnormalities, a large intake of caffeine may aggravate these symptoms. This small percentage of people would be wise to severely limit their caffeine consumption.

* Can drinking coffee aggravate my mild hypertension?

Until quite recently our answer would have been "yes." A research study had shown that blood pressure was increased in persons with borderline high blood pressure after taking the equivalent caffeine in two to three cups of coffee. The blood pressure peak at one hour was enough to cause a false-positive diagnosis of hypertension. But as with much research, we must look closer.

In this study the volunteers had abstained from caffeine for three weeks prior to the test and consequently may have been more sensitive to a caffeine load. Further studies on people who drank caffeine-containing beverages daily, showed that drinking two to three cups of coffee at one sitting did not increase blood pressure. Apparently regular users adapt to caffeine's effects and their blood pressure is not elevated after a moderate amount is taken.

It should be noted that a small percentage of people are exceptionally sensitive to the effects of caffeine. Their blood pressure as well as other body processes will react adversely to a caffeine load. As they age, this sensitivity will increase, particularly with regard to blood pressure.

If you are hypertensive, moderate caffeine consumption should be safe. It would be wise, however, not to overuse caffeine, as an excessive intake might be reflected in your blood pressure reading. (For additional information on hypertension see Chapter 8.)

* Is it true that drinking too much coffee can cause cystitis?

Yes, an excessive coffee or tea intake can cause cystitis, an inflammation of the urinary bladder. This type of cystitis is not caused by an infection but by the diuretic effect of coffee and tea resulting in excessive urination and irritation to the urethra. The inflammation is temporary, lasting only a day or two, and is not harmful to your health.

* I enjoy drinking coffee but I have heard that the caffeine in it can cause breast lumps. Is this true?

It may be hard to give up your cup of coffee, but in a group of women with benign lumps who did just that, the incidence of lumps was markedly reduced. Recent evidence suggests there is a relationship between the consumption of methylated xanthines (caffeine is one) and benign breast lumps, also called "fibrocystic breast disease." Other methylated xanthines to avoid are theophylline (found in tea) and theobromine (found in cocoa and cola). Women with benign breast lumps are advised to limit their use of these foods. (For a more detailed explanation of fibrocystic breast disease see Chapter 5.)

* Will switching to decaffeinated coffee relieve my heartburn?

If you are bothered by chronic heartburn you should eliminate all coffee rather than switch to decaffeinated. Heartburn, which has nothing to do with the heart, occurs when acidic stomach contents splash back and up into the tender lining of the esophagus, resulting in burning and pain.

We know now that both coffee and decaffeinated coffee, as well as tea, increase the acidity of the stomach and relax muscles in this area, allowing back-splashing into the esophagus. Something in coffee and tea other than caffeine is causing this.

To help control heartburn, avoid all coffee, tea, and highly spiced foods while eating small frequent meals. The small meals prevent the stomach from becoming too full and lessen the possible backup of its contents into the esophagus.

Ulcer sufferers may also find all coffee irritating since it causes excess stomach acid. If coffee aggravates ulcers, it was speculated, coffee might have caused the ulcer to form in the first place. This is false. Two investigations studied the role of coffee as a cause of ulcers in more than sixty thousand people and no significant risk was found.

* Will drinking decaffeinated coffee increase my chances of getting cancer?

In this issue coffee is not the culprit, but the solvent used to decaffeinate the coffee may be. General Foods had at one time used trichloroethylene (TCE) to extract the caffeine from the coffee beans in their Sanka and Brim coffees. TCE in large doses causes liver cancer in mice. With these findings in mind, General Foods voluntarily switched to methylene chloride for the extraction process in the late 1970s.

Those of you with a history of drinking Brim or Sanka may be wondering about the fate of your liver. Relax. To match the test doses of TCE fed to the mice, you would have to drink 50 million cups of the coffee a day for life.

Methylene chloride, currently used as the decaffeinating solvent, is an FDA-approved food additive, but the National Cancer Institute, noting that it is a member of a suspect group of chlorinated hydrocarbons, is doing studies on the safety of its use.

Specialty food shops in major cities may be a source of a Swiss imported decaffeinated coffee in which the caffeine is extracted by a water-solvent process. Although expensive, this coffee is free of chemical residue.

ALCOHOL

* What happens to alcohol in my body?

Alcohol requires no digestion and can be absorbed throughout your digestive tract. The blood can hold large amounts, causing a depression of the central nervous system resulting in a series of effects. First, judgment, coordination, walking, and speech are impaired. Next, emotions, memory, and reflexes are affected. At this point, you are drunk and unable to walk or talk straight. If drinking continues, stupor and coma may result.

Alcohol is toxic, a poison to the body, attacking the liver, heart, digestive tract, pancreas, and bone marrow. It was once believed a good diet with ample protein could prevent the damage of excessive drinking, but we now know proper food cannot prevent the progressive poisoning of alcohol.

Ninety percent of all alcohol consumed reaches the liver, which must break it down and excrete it. Alcohol, however, interferes with liver function, and with excessive drinking the liver may be damaged beyond repair. No matter how much alcohol is consumed, the liver can handle only *one ounce per hour*. Two martinis will take three hours to clear the system—no faster, no slower, unaffected by exercise, black coffee, or a cold shower.

✻ How many calories are there in a Manhattan?

Alcoholic beverages are often referred to as "empty calorie" foods, not because they lack calories but because they contribute little to the diet except calories. Beer contains niacin, as does wine, which also has small amounts of other B vitamins (thiamine, riboflavin, B_6, and pantothenic acid) and iron. Other vitamins and minerals are present in trace amounts or not at all. (See the chart "Calories in Alcoholic Drinks.")

✻ When I drink a martini, how much alcohol am I getting?

The proof on alcoholic beverages is not the actual percentage of alcohol in that bottle. If something is 80 proof it is 40 percent alcohol; the proof is double the percentage of alcohol. This, however, still does not tell you how many ounces of pure alcohol you are drinking. A simple calculation to determine this is to multiply .08 by the number of drinks you had. For example: .08 × 3 beers = 2.4, or approximately 2½ ounces of alcohol. The multiplication factor of .08 is an average figure based on standard drink sizes: a 1½-ounce jigger, 12-ounce can of beer, and 4-ounce glass of wine.

A martini is a jigger and a half of gin plus a half-jigger of vermouth, totaling 3 ounces or equal to two drinks. Therefore, .08 × 2 = 1.6, or there is slightly more than 1½ ounces of alcohol in a regular martini.

CALORIES IN SOME ALCOHOLIC DRINKS

Drink	Size	Calories
Ale	1 mug (12 ounces)	148
Beer	1 mug (12 ounces)	173
Beer, Light	1 mug (12 ounces)	90
Cognac	1 brandy glass (2 ounces)	150
Cordials		
Anisette	1 cordial glass (1½ ounces)	150
Apricot brandy	1 cordial glass (1½ ounces)	130
Crème de menthe	1 cordial glass (1½ ounces)	136
Curaçao	1 cordial glass (1½ ounces)	110
Daiquiri	1 cocktail (3½ ounces)	124
Gin	1 jigger (1½ ounces)	107
Manhattan	1 cocktail (3½ ounces)	167
Martini	1 cocktail (3½ ounces)	143
Old-fashioned	1 glass (4 ounces)	183
Rum	1 jigger (1½ ounces)	107
Rye	1 jigger (1½ ounces)	122
Scotch	1 jigger (1½ ounces)	107
Tom Collins	1 cocktail (10 ounces)	182
Wine, port	1 wineglass (4 ounces)	193
Wine, red	1 wineglass (4 ounces)	83
Wine, sauterne	1 wineglass (4 ounces)	97

* Does alcohol contain an anti-aging factor?

We wouldn't go that far, but the idea that alcohol can extend our life-span may not be farfetched. Our Puritan ethic makes us suspicious of the idea that if something is enjoyable it can also be good for us. But the best available evidence indicates that those who drink with moderation live longer, on the average, than those who abstain or drink lightly (less than one drink a day). Further, moderate drinkers live longer than heavy drinkers (in excess of two drinks daily) or former drinkers. Isn't it nice to know that in the quest for good health *all* of life's pleasures need not be cast aside?

* Is a drink before bed better than a sleeping pill?

A glass of wine is often recommended as a mild sedative. The calming effect you feel is not from the alcohol but from *congeners,* secondary products formed during fermentation, found in wine. Congeners not only calm you but inhibit the absorption of alcohol into your bloodstream while enhancing the absorption of calcium, phosphorus, magnesium, zinc, and iron.

The question is, should you be taking the wine just before you go to sleep? Yes, if you limit it to one small glass. Even moderate amounts of alcohol interfere with REM sleep, a normal deep sleep cycle that is necessary to feeling completely rested.

Many people find a glass of wine or a small cordial relaxing and this amount could certainly be used safely to induce sleep.

* Will a drink before dinner cause me to eat more?

Moderate amounts of alcohol do have an appetite-stimulating effect that will last about fifteen to twenty minutes. A drink before dinner most certainly adds to the enjoyment of the meal, and although it makes you eager to eat, there is no proof that the drink encourages you to overeat.

As a matter of fact, wine has been recommended in weight-control programs. The calming effect may reduce the emotional tension that often causes overeating. This relaxes the person so that he eats more slowly. One study showed that overweight people ate less when wine was drunk along with the meal.

Just keep in mind that alcoholic beverages have calories, so drinks before or with dinner should be kept to only a few. As with most things in life, moderation is important.

* I often feel obliged to have a drink when I'm out socially. What should I order?

We know how you feel. Sometimes it is difficult and awkward not to take a drink. The trick is to drink during a meal, in order to interfere with the absorption of the alcohol into your body. When alcohol is taken on an empty stomach, the highest blood alcohol peaks are caused by gin, vodka, and whiskey, followed by dessert wines, sherry, and vermouth. The alcohol in table wines and beer are the least efficiently absorbed into your bloodstream.

Alcohol rapidly enters the bloodstream from the digestive tract and as the blood alcohol concentration increases, so do the symptoms you feel. One drink (blood alcohol of .02) and you're relaxed. Ten drinks (blood alcohol of .20) and you're legally drunk with erratic emotions and lack of coordination.

When alcoholic beverages are coupled with a meal, absorption into the bloodstream is sharply reduced. This suggests that you should drink *with* a meal rather than *before* and that beer or table wine are your best choices. Remember, too, that mineral water with lime is an "in" drink.

* Can wine "thicken" my blood?

For years, it has been a common assumption that "red" wines, especially port, were useful to *strengthen* the blood and cure anemia. Actually, table wine, both red and white, has more iron than port. A 4-ounce glass provides a man or post-menopausal woman with about 5 percent of his or her daily need. You'd need to drink over 3 quarts of wine a day if your goal was to get *all* your iron from wine!

* What's in alcohol that protects drinkers from heart disease?

The heart appears to benefit from moderate amounts of alcohol. One to two drinks a day (a drink being 1½ ounces of distilled liquor, 12 ounces of beer, or 5 ounces of table wine) has been linked to a *decreased* risk of coronary death. The effect, however, is only apparent in light drinkers. Heavy drinkers do not have the same decreased risk.

Among heavy drinkers, high blood pressure, abnormal heart rhythms, and cardiomyopathy (a type of heart disease) are common. Death due to heart disease is not unusual at a relatively early age.

How does alcohol protect against heart disease? The theory is that moderate drinking increases the body's level of high-density lipoproteins (HDL). These complex blood proteins are believed to protect against heart disease and those with higher levels of HDL are at lowered risk. Further, small doses of alcohol—one drink—have a calming effect; perhaps this helps the heart by reducing stress. (See Chapter 8, for more information on heart disease.)

✳ Can I have an occasional drink if I'm on a low-sodium diet?

Most wines contain less than 20 milligrams of sodium in a 5-ounce glass and are certainly acceptable on a low-sodium diet. Hard alcohol (gin, Scotch, vodka, etc.) has virtually no sodium. The sodium in beer is dependent on the sodium concentration in the brewery water supply; many brands have low concentrations.

A note of caution: If you are taking any medication for high blood pressure or heart rhythm problems, remember alcohol and drugs *don't mix!*

✳ My wife won't let me have my evening highball now that I'm taking medicine for high blood pressure. Isn't she wrong?

As a rule, alcohol and drugs shouldn't be taken together. Although interactions are predictable, the intensity of the reaction varies markedly from one person to another and from one occasion to another.

The liver metabolizes both drugs and alcohol. When alcohol is present, liver activity is increased and drugs may be metabolized more quickly, reducing their effectiveness. If large amounts are drunk, the alcohol may block the normal drug metabolism and prolong its activity in the body. In extreme situations drug toxicity can result. (See the chart "Alcohol + Drugs = Danger." Note the reaction with high blood pressure medication.)

* As a diabetic, can't I have an occasional glass of wine or a beer?

If you are taking oral antidiabetic drugs the answer is no. If you control your diabetes by diet or diet and insulin injections, the answer is a guarded yes.

European physicians have always allowed diabetics to drink dry table wines. Physicians in the United States usually discourage this. Since diabetes is characterized by an inability to utilize carbohydrates properly, it follows that alcoholic beverages included in the diet must be low in sugar and other carbohydrates. Dry red wine and dry white wine contain less than ⅛ teaspoon (0.2 to 0.4 gram) sugar in a 4-ounce serving. Dry rosé and dry champagne have about ⅓ teaspoon (1.3 to 1.8 grams) sugar in a 4-ounce serving. Dry sherry has the highest sugar content, having the equivalent of a ½ teaspoon (2.4 grams) sugar in 4 ounces. A serving of any of these could be enjoyed by a diabetic. Sweet dessert and kosher wines should not be used because they are too high in sugar.

Beer and "light" beer have more sugar and carbohydrate and need to be used more sparingly. A 12-ounce glass of beer has 13.7 grams of carbohydrate, the equivalent of 2¾ teaspoons sugar. Light beer is a better choice, having 5.5 grams in 12 ounces or the equivalent of slightly more than 1 teaspoon sugar. A "nip"—a 6-to-8-ounce serving of light beer—would be equal to drinking a glass of dry sherry.

Distilled spirits—vodka, gin, Scotch, rye—contain no sugar, it has all been fermented to alcohol.

If your diabetes is under control, you can safely have a drink occasionally. Alcohol calories could be substituted for an equal number of fat calories in your daily food plan. It's a trade-off: wine with dinner but no butter on your bread.

* Does alcohol cause cancer?

Alcohol, by itself, does not *cause* cancer but it does appear to *promote* cancers caused by other factors. This risk is most dramatic for those who drink more than moderate amounts and smoke. Large amounts of alcohol impair immunological responses, increasing susceptibility to infection and possibly cancer. Cancers of the mouth and throat are two to six times more common among heavy drinkers than nondrinkers, and heavy drinking plus smoking raises the risk fifteen times. Similar risks exist for cancers of the larynx (voice box) and esophagus.

One study found a strong relationship between deaths from rectal cancer and the amount of beer consumed. Beer and Scotch whiskey, both made from malt, contain N-nitroso-dimethylamine or NDMA, one of a family of carcinogens called "nitrosamines."

The liver, the only organ in the body capable of metabolizing alcohol, is also extremely suspectible to alcohol damage. An injured liver may be unable to detoxify carcinogens that find their way into the body. Cancer of the liver is common among alcoholics.

* Today at lunch I was told to skip the wine because I'm taking an antibiotic. Why?

You were given good advice. People who are taking general antibiotics—Amcill, Omnipen, Polycillin, and Principen—may become ill if they drink alcohol. The reaction may consist of flushing, pounding heartbeat, shortness of breath, dizziness, and weakness. Remember a strong dose of a cough/cold remedy could trigger the same reaction. Most drugs simply don't mix with alcohol. (See the following question and the chart "Alcohol + Drugs = Danger.")

* Do most cold remedies contain alcohol?

Not only cold remedies but vitamin tonics and iron supplements as well. Alcohol is the dilutant in over five-hundred medications, frequently found in "elixirs" and "tonics."

The alcohol in one drug can interact with another drug, causing serious consequences. Two tablespoons of a cough/

cold remedy with 25 percent alcohol is a 50-proof medicine equivalent to 5 ounces of wine. A dose of this, mixed with a dose of Miltown, a mild tranquilizer, will markedly increase the sedative effect and may cause serious central nervous system depression. Combined with a high blood pressure medication like Aldomet, it can cause a blood pressure drop that is dangerously low.

Alcohol in medications is not innocuous. The chart "Alcohol in Medications" will alert you to the products that should be used only when you are not taking other drugs. If you are on regular medication, consult your doctor before using an alcohol-containing drug. The proof is double the alcohol percent: a 10 percent alcohol solution is 20 proof; a 20 percent alcohol solution is 40 proof, and so on. Some of these medications can pack quite a wallop, so be careful.

DRUGS

✳ Does what I eat affect the medication I take?

Most definitely. An asthma sufferer can reduce his or her medication's effectiveness by over 50 percent after a few charcoal-broiled summer meals. Taking antibiotics with milk or a meal may be the reason that an infection just won't clear up. Coumadin often is prescribed for phlebitis and stroke patients, to "thin" their blood and prevent clot formation. The medication's effect may be reduced by eating broccoli, beef liver, cabbage, lettuce, spinach, and asparagus. All these foods are high in vitamin K, the nutrient needed for normal blood clotting. When these are eaten often by someone taking Coumadin, the level of vitamin K in the body increases beyond the point where the medication can counteract it and life-threatening clots may form.

If you have been directed to take your medication on an empty stomach, do so. Take the medicine one hour before meals or two hours after eating, using a large glassful of water to wash it down. (See the chart "Drugs to Take on an Empty Stomach.")

ALCOHOL IN MEDICATIONS

Drug	Percent of alcohol content
Benadryl Elixir	14.0
Benylin Cough Syrup	5.0
Breacol (metholated)	20.0
Breacol (regular formula)	10.0
Broncho-Tussin	40.0
Cheracol Syrup	3.0
Chlotrimetron	7.0
Comtrex Nighttime Multi Symptom	25.0
Co-Tylenol Liquid Cough Formula	7.0
Dimetapp Elixir	2.3
Dramamine Liquid	5.0
Dristan Cough Formula	12.0
Eldertonic	15.0
Feosol Elixir	5.0
Geritol	12.0
Lomotil Liquid	15.0
Nembutal Elixir	18.0
Neo-Synephrine	8.0
Novahistine DMX	10.0
Nyquil	25.0
Pertussin 8-Hour Cough Formula	9.5
Pertussin Plus Night-Time Cold Medicine	25.0
Quibron Elixir	15.0
Robitussin	3.5
Romilar CF	10.0
Stannitol Elixir	23.0
Triaminic Expectorant	5.0
Tylenol Liquid	7.0
Vick's Formula 44	10.0

ALCOHOL + DRUGS = DANGER

Combination	May cause . . .
Alcohol + aspirin Alka-Seltzer Bufferin Excedrin	stomach irritation, gastrointestinal bleeding

Combination	May cause . . .
Alcohol + nonnarcotic pain-killers Datril Bromo-Seltzer Tylenol	stomach irritation, gastrointestinal bleeding, liver damage
Alcohol + antihistamines Allerest Contac Dramamine Dristan	increased central nervous system depression, drowsiness
Alcohol + narcotic pain killers Codeine Darvon	increased central nervous system depression with acute intoxication, possible respiratory arrest
Alcohol + high blood pressure medication Aldomet Dyazide Lasix	increased effect, in some cases blood pressure can be lowered to dangerous levels, increased intoxication
Alcohol + anticoagulants Coumadin Dicumarol	increased or decreased effect
Alcohol + oral antidiabetic drugs Diabinese Orinase	decreased antidiabetic effect, flushing, severe headache, pounding heartbeat, dizziness, shortness of breath, sweating, initial rise in blood pressure, weakness nausea, vomiting
Alcohol + antibiotics Amcill Omnipen Polycillin	reaction similar to that seen with oral antidiabetic drugs
Alcohol + sedatives or tranquilizers Valium Librium Miltown	increased sedative effect, increased central nervous system depression; combination could be lethal

Combination	May cause . . .
Alcohol + antidepressants Aventyl Elavil Norpramin Sinequan	extreme increases in blood pressure, excessive sedation, incoordination, stomach upset; combination could be lethal

Drugs to Take on an Empty Stomach

Drug	Classification
Achromycin*†	antibiotic
Aminophylline, theophylline, Slo-Phyllin	bronchodilators
Ampicillin	antiinfection
Castor oil‡	laxative
Cuprimine	antiarthritic
Declomycin (demeclocycline)*†	antiinfection
Epsom salts‡	laxative
Erythromycin*	antiinfective
Fleet	laxative
Gantrisin	urinary antiinfective
Gaviscon	antacid
Gelusil	antacid
Librax	antispasmodic
Mylanta	antacid
Penicillamine	antiarthritic
Penicillin*	antiinfective
Pronestyl	antiarrhythmic
Quinidex	antiarrhythmic
Somophyllin	bronchodilator
Tetracycline†	antiinfective
Theo-Dur, Theolair	bronchodilator
Tylenol	analgesic
Vibramycin (doxycycline)*†	antiinfective

* Fruit juice, vegetable juice, soda pop, and wine are all acidic drinks and will reduce the effectiveness of antibiotics.

† Avoid milk and dairy products; they will reduce effectiveness.

‡ Take with juice.

✳ My prescription for Motrin says "take with meals." Why?

Many drugs are terribly irritating and when taken on an empty stomach may cause pain, nausea, vomiting, and diar-

106

rhea. Arthritis medications, like Motrin, are less irritating if taken with food.

Other drugs like Aldactone for high blood pressure should be taken with meals so that they are absorbed.

"With meals," means just before, during, or immediately after eating. (See the chart "Drugs to Take with Meals.")

DRUGS TO TAKE WITH MEALS

Drug	Classification
Aldactone	antihypertension
Aldoril	antihypertension
Aspirin	analgesic
Butazolidin	antiarthritic
Colace	laxative
Darvon Compound	analgesic
Diuril	antihypertensive
Dramamine	antiemetic (motion sickness)
Empirin Compound (with codeine)	analgesic
Feosol*	iron supplement
Fer-In-Sol*	iron supplement
Flagyl	antiinfection
Fulvicin	antiinfection
Grifulvin	antiinfection
Inderal	antihypertensive, antimigraine
Indocin	antiarthritic
Kaochlor	potassium supplement
Lithane†	tranquilizer
Mellaril	tranquilizer
Mortrin	antiarthritic
Oretic	antihypertensive
Ornade	antihistaminic
Premarin	hormone (estrogen)
Sinemet	antiparkinsonian
Sinequan	antidepressant
Tagamet	antiulcer
Tandearil	antiinflammatory

Drug	Classification
Thorazine	tranquilizer
Triavil	antidepressant
Valium	antianxiety
Zyloprim	antigout

* Do not take with milk; use a fruit juice high in vitamin C.
† Take with milk.

* If I'm taking medication for a long time should I take a multivitamin?

Drugs frequently interfere with nutrient absorption. We've already mentioned the interaction of vitamin K and anticoagulants (see the question "Does what I eat effect the medication I take?" earlier in this section) as well as the interaction of antacids with mineral absorption (see question "Which is the best antacid to use?" in this section). If you regularly take medication, we'd recommend a daily adult multivitamin-mineral supplement such as Centrum or One-A-Day Vitamins Plus Minerals.

* Now that I'm over sixty I notice a stronger reaction to some drugs. Why?

Your reaction to a drug and its effectiveness in your body is dependent on many things: whether your stomach is full or empty; whether you're taking other drugs; what your state of health is; and most importantly, your age.

We're not suggesting sixty is old, but a sixty-year-old body, regardless of how vigorous, will react differently to drugs from a thirty-year-old body. Even though you may be unaware of it, your body has slowed down. This will affect your ability to handle drugs—absorption, metabolism, transportation, and excretion.

Your stomach is less acidic, your heart is not pumping as vigorously, some blood vessels may be congested, and the amount of muscle and water in your body has decreased. All this affects drug absorption and transportation. The liver, which breaks down drugs, and the kidney, which eliminates drugs, are both working more slowly, hence drugs may be broken down and excreted more slowly. They stay in the system longer. This can lead to an adverse drug reaction.

Generally, we are more sensitive to drugs as we get older and can achieve the same effect with a smaller dose. If you are experiencing any unusual "feeling" from medication you regularly take, discuss this with your doctor so he or she can make necessary adjustments.

* I am taking a diuretic, do I need a potassium supplement?

Diuretics are used to rid the body of excess sodium and fluid. Many of them cause potassium loss as well, and in that situation there is an increased need for potassium. Many people taking these diuretics can get all the potassium they need from food, without the need for a supplement. While there is no way to estimate how much additional potassium an individual will need, a committee of the National Research Council recently suggested that about 3,900 milligrams would be a reasonable amount. After a few weeks on a diuretic, a simple blood test to check serum potassium level shows if the person is taking in enough potassium to make up for the loss from the diuretic.

Potassium can come from a variety of sources—prune juice, orange juice, bananas, potatoes, lentils, and beans are good because they are also low in sodium, and you are probably trying to restrict that also. Other usual foods such as milk, meat, bread, and cereals are good sources of potassium too. Some people use salt substitutes that contain potassium. Ask your doctor about these or potassium preparations such as K-Lyte/Cl, or Kaochlor.

Any of the following will supply about 500 milligrams of potassium.

1 medium banana	1¼ cups orange juice
1¼ cups grapefruit juice	1 cup prune juice
½ cantaloupe	1 large white or sweet potato
⅓ cup lentils	¾ cup kidney beans

See Chapter 8 for additional information and the chart "Sodium and Potassium in Foods."

* Which is the best antacid to use?

Antacids are commonly taken by large numbers of people. Aggressive advertisements have led us to believe that we are constantly fighting a battle against acidity, and if we lose, we suffer. Hence, millions take antacids daily without giving the drug a second thought. They should, since the natural strong acidity of the stomach is a desirable condition. Systemic antacids attempt to neutralize the naturally acidic stomach contents. Even if they are only partially successful this disturbs the body's balance system.

Calcium carbonate antacids (Tums) are quite effective, but when used habitually they result in severe constipation. The constipation is rarely linked to the antacid but presumed to be a natural consequence of "indigestion."

Antacids with aluminum hydroxide bind with phosphates in the body and prevent phosphate absorption. If the antacid is overused, bone absorption of phosphate may be virtually blocked leading to a bone disease called "osteomalacia." (See Chapter 5 for more information on bone disease.) Iron is absorbed poorly when antacids lower the stomach's acidity, and thiamine, a B vitamin, is destroyed when antacids follow a meal. By decreasing the acidity of the stomach, antacids react with drugs. Some drugs will be absorbed more quickly while others may never reach therapeutic levels. Those influenced by antacid ingestion include: aspirin, Digoxin, Indocin, Mellaril, Inderal, and tetracycline antibiotics. (See Chapter 6 for suggestions on how to deal with indigestion.)

Note: If you regularly use antacids they may add a significant amount of sodium to your diet. (One Rolaids tablet has 53 milligrams of sodium. See Chapter 8 for more information on the sodium content of antacids, and see Chapter 6 for more information on antacids.)

* I am taking thyroid medication. I was told not to eat a lot of cabbage, Brussels sprouts, or cauliflower. Why?

Cabbage, Brussels sprouts, and cauliflower (also broccoli, kale, kohlrabi, rutabagas, turnips, mustard greens, and soybean products) all contain antithyroid substances called "goitrogens." These goitrogens act on the thyroid gland and prevent it from making thyroid hormone. There is the possibility that eating large quantities of these vegetables could interfere with the medication you take. Be sure to eat only moderate amounts.

* My friend recommended Gerovital H₃ to slow down many of the effects of aging. How much should I use?

Professor Ana Aslan of the Bucharest Institute has been proclaiming Gerovital H_3 as "the secret of eternal vigor and youth" for over thirty years. Advocates claim it prevents or relieves heart disease, arthritis, deafness, Parkinson's disease, senile psychoses, high blood pressure, wrinkling, psoriasis, anxiety, peptic ulcers, and impotence. If that isn't enough—it's also supposed to stimulate hair growth and restore your hair's natural color.

Does it work? After extensive review, Dr. Ostfeld of Yale University School of Medicine says no. Gerovital is procaine, the generic name for Novocain. Sound familiar? It should to anyone who has ever visited the dentist. Gerovital is nothing more than a local anesthetic. There is some evidence that Gerovital H_3 may work as an antidepressant, but there are other more effective medications that can be used.

A note of caution: Although side effects are rare, some people may be allergic to procaine, experiencing low blood pressure, breathing difficulties, flushing, itching, skin rash, and possibly convulsions.

* I am taking Lithane (lithium) for depression. Does it have any effect on what I eat?

So far as we know, lithium is not an essential nutrient. It is used as a drug to prevent recurrent attacks of certain mental disorders.

When you take Lithane, Lithotabs, or Lithonate, you have an increased need for sodium to prevent any toxic effects from the drug. Any person on a low-sodium diet who is also taking lithium should consult his or her doctor about this. It's also wise to limit caffeine-containing foods, drink large amounts of water (two to three quarts) each day, and take your required dose with a meal or with a large glass of milk.

✻ Is it true that I should not eat aged cheese if I'm taking an antidepressant drug?

That depends on what drug you are taking. A group of drugs called "monoamine oxidase inhibitiors" (MAOIs) react very dramatically with certain foods and can precipitate a high blood pressure crisis. Once commonplace, MAOIs have by and large been replaced with other antidepressant drugs. Some MAOIs—Parnate, Eutonyl, and Nardil—are still in use.

MAOIs react with foods containing tyramine. Aged cheese is the worst offender but many additional foods must be avoided as well. These include:

Avocados

Bananas

Beer

Bologna

Canned figs

Cheese-containing foods
(like casseroles)

Chianti wine

Chocolate

Dates

Liver

Meat extracts (like Marmite
and Bovril)

Meat tenderizers

Nuts

Papaya

Patés

Pickled and kippered herring

Pepperoni

Raisins

Salami

Sausage

Soups (canned and instant)

Sour cream

Soy sauce

Yeast or yeast extracts

Yogurt

MAOI drugs also interact with other drugs—diet pills, high blood pressure regulators, insulin, and oral anti-diabetic medications.

Since the reactions caused are so acute, patients need careful counseling by their doctor and the motivaton to strictly follow an all-fresh-food diet.

5

For Women Only

Women are members of one of the fastest growing segments of the population. There are presently 43,642 million women over the age of forty in the United States—19.6 percent of the total population. Projections indicate that by the year 2000, one out of every fourteen Americans will be a woman over sixty-five. Today's woman has so many options: she can be a career woman, homemaker, mother, student, volunteer, or a combination of these (maybe all of them!). No one works harder than a woman who has a job (paid or not) and the responsibilities of a home and a family. All that activity calls for a healthy, well-nourished body to cope with the stress and strain of daily life.

You are concerned about your health and well-being. A 1980 survey showed 50 percent of women in the United States had a greater interest in nutrition now as compared to three years before. You are trying to exercise more and eat foods that will help you to maintain good health and see you through your busy days. Further, you hope the changes you are making now will postpone or eliminate health problems as years pass. As nutritionists, and women, we are convinced that nutrition—what you eat—can greatly influence your health now and your well-being in the future.

As women, our nutritional needs are often different from men's. By virtue of a smaller body size, we need to take in approximately the same amount of nutrients in fewer calories and often we have smaller body nutrient reserves to draw

113

upon if needed. Women also face more nutritionally demanding episodes in life than do men. Each month, until menopause, about 15 milligrams of iron are lost in menstruation, which must be replaced to prevent anemia. Pregnancy, breast feeding, even using oral contraceptives, compromises our nutritional well-being. Often we reach middle age nutritionally depleted, increasing our susceptibility to osteoporosis and the stresses of menopause.

But wait. This gloomy picture need not be so. A well-nourished woman easily replaces her monthly iron loss, nourishes her fetus and her own body, and handles the nutritional side effects of oral contraceptives with little difficulty. Good nutrition will see you through menopause, relieving many symptoms. Osteoporosis need not be inevitable. Adequate exercise, calcium, vitamin D, and fluoride should keep your bones healthy and strong till ninety!

At forty, a woman has truly reached her prime and good nutrition can help her to enjoy it to the fullest. A quote from Margaret Mead is worth keeping in mind as you pass through this next stage in your life: "The most creative force in the world is a menopausal woman with zest."

✱ Are all women anemic?

Estimates suggest that forty percent of all adult women under fifty show indications of iron deficiency. Menstrual blood loss and the drain of pregnancy make it difficult for a woman to maintain her iron reserves. Iron-deficient blood cells are smaller and lighter in color than normal. They are unable to carry enough oxygen throughout the body, and you are left feeling fatigued, weak, and suffering from headaches.

The RDA for iron is 18 milligrams a day for women under fifty. The average American diet usually falls short of this need. The following sample diet illustrates this clearly and suggests that most women would benefit from a daily iron supplement.

See the chart "Iron in Foods" in the Minerals section of Chapter 2 for a list of food sources of iron.

Remember: Tea, milk, cereal, and eggs reduce iron ab-

MEETING A WOMAN'S IRON NEEDS THROUGH FOOD

Food	Portion	Milligrams of iron
Cornflakes	1 cup	0.5
Toast	1 slice	0.6
Orange juice	½ cup	0.3
Roast beef sandwich	1	4.1
Potato chips	1 ounce	0.6
Banana	1 medium	0.8
Milk	1 cup	0.1
Chicken, fried	¼	1.8
Potato	1 small	0.5
Green beans	½ cup	0.4
Applesauce	½ cup	0.6
Corn muffin	1	0.6
TOTAL		10.9

sorption in the body. Orange juice and other foods high in vitamin C improve absorption. Your iron supplement will be absorbed better if you take it with a meal containing meat and a source of vitamin C.

* If I'm on the "pill" does it affect my nutrition?

The nutritional influence of oral contraceptives is different for each woman depending on the type of pill used, her age, the length of pill use, and her state of nutrition before use. Older women who have had many pregnancies and eat an inadequate diet have the greatest risk for a "borderline" nutrient deficiency.

The effect of oral contraceptives on nutrition is getting a lot of attention. The "pill" alters body levels of several nutrients. Nutrient levels are generally measured by serum (blood) values. We have normal blood values for most nutrients and we compare the nutrient blood values of pill users against these.

The blood values change in pill users. Serum levels of B_6, folic acid, and vitamin C go down. Lowered, but less significantly, are levels of B$_{12}$, thiamine, and riboflavin. Blood values for iron, vitamin A, and copper increase. Seems simple. If blood values go down we should supplement with those nutrients in short supply. If blood values increase there is no need for supplementation. Unfortunately, that is not the case. What appears simple is, in fact, quite complicated.

For example, it was believed for some time that pill users needed less vitamin A because their blood levels showed higher than normal amounts. What was actually happening was that the oral contraceptive had the ability to draw vitamin A out of storage in the liver and put the vitamin into circulation in the blood. This gave high blood levels but low body stores of the vitamin. It looked as if the women needed *less* vitamin A when in actuality they needed *more* to replace lost body stores. The same effect occurs with copper.

Nutrition information for pill users is scanty. Some authorities believe firmly in supplementation while others feel a varied, balanced diet is all the insurance a pill user needs. Until all the research is in, we feel a daily supplement of a multivitamin-mineral preparation with amounts close to the RDA is a good idea. Pill users have been diagnosed as deficient in folic acid and a significant, though small, percentage are marginally low in B$_6$.

The one nutrient bonus that is certain for pill users is that they will have an increase in the body's iron stores. This is due to a reduced menstrual blood loss and an increased iron-binding capacity. (See the question "Which vitamin should I take to relieve my feelings of depression?" later in this chapter for more information on vitamin-oral contraceptive interaction.)

BREAST PROBLEMS

✳ Can eliminating coffee reduce my breast lumps?

We feel pretty strongly that it can. However, coffee is not the villain, caffeine is. Or even more correctly, fibrocystic breast disease, which afflicts over one-third of all American women, may be affected by the consumption of methylated xanthines.

The issue is complicated so we'll go over it very carefully. Fibrocystic breast disease is characterized by cyclic pain and swelling of the breasts brought about by the growth of fibrous tissue and accumulation of fluid-filled cysts in the breasts. For many women the condition causes persistent breast lumps and pain. The lumps may be so extensive that they mask any tumor growth in the breast and make regular breast examinations difficult.

In 1979, Dr. John Minton published results of an experiment linking the consumption of methylated xanthines to the aggravation of fibrocystic breast disease. Methylated xanthines are a group of stimulants, of which caffeine is one. Theophylline, found in tea, and theobromine in chocolate are also part of this group.

Minton worked with twenty women who eliminated all methylxanthine–containing foods from their diets. This means no coffee, no tea, no cola, orange, or lemon-lime soda, and no chocolate-flavored foods. (See Chapter 4 for a complete list of caffeine-containing foods and medications.) For seventeen of the twenty women in this study the breast lumps disappeared. If the woman smoked, the lumps took longer to disappear, but the condition did clear up. Older women needed to stay with the elimination diet for a longer period to gain relief. This could suggest a cumulative effect from chronic methylxanthine consumption.

This research does not conclusively prove a cause-and-effect relationship between breast lumps and methylated xanthines. It will take definitive research and many years to prove Minton's theory. In the meantime, however, for women who suffer from fibrocystic breast disease, there can be no harm done if they abstain from coffee, tea, cola, and drugs containing methylated xanthines. (See the following questions on breast disease for further information.)

* If I have fibrocystic breast disease, does that mean I can never drink regular coffee again?

It might. We have counseled many women regarding the elimination of caffeine and related compounds from their diet. Each person reacted individually. In all cases the women experienced relief from the cystic breast disease; however, some seemed far more sensitive to methylated xanthines than others.

In one case, the woman just cut out cola beverages (she had been drinking six to eight a day) and caffeine-containing medications and continued to drink one or two cups of coffee or tea a day. Within a month, she reported being able "to sleep on my stomach for the first time in years." The symptoms never returned as long as she continued her moderate elimination.

In another case, the sensitivity was so great that decaffeinated coffee (containing a few milligrams of caffeine) and cocoa (also low in caffeine) were enough to cause symptoms. This woman had to *totally* eliminate all methylated xanthine–containing food and even the most innocent "cheating" resulted in a recurrence of pain.

If you have removed all of the offending foods from your diet and have experienced relief from symptoms, you may be able to add some foods back. Some women can adjust their methylated xanthine consumption to a level, such as one cup of coffee a day, where the disease is not symptomatic.

✳ My friend is taking vitamin E to treat her breast lumps, is this a good idea?

We have seen this approach work in treating fibrocystic breast disease. Vitamin E therapy eliminates the symptoms, it does not eliminate the breast lumps.

The treatment is based on the work of Dr. Robert London, who found that vitamin E supplementation relieves the symptoms of cystic breast disease and in some women reduced the size of the breast lumps. Dr. London suggests 600 I.U. vitamin E daily for eight weeks. About half the women treated had tremendous relief from pain and swelling.

✳ Is cystic breast disease a cancerous condition?

Fibrocystic breast disease is a benign condition—*not* cancerous. However, those women who have cystic breast disease may have a greater risk of having breast cancer in the future. Therefore, cystic breast disease needs to be considered as a risk factor—one of many.

Other risk factors for breast cancer are:

- *Age.* The longer a woman lives the more likely she is to develop breast cancer. It kills more women than any other cancer and kills more women age forty to forty-four than any other disease.

- *Genetics.* The risks increase if a grandmother or mother had breast cancer. Jewish women of European descent are at slightly greater risk than any other subgroup.

- *Reproductive history.* Those with early menarche and late menopause are at greatest risk.

- *Hormone activity.* The use of oral contraceptives or estrogen replacement therapy increases risk.

- *Exposure to ionizing radiation.* Excessive X rays may increase risk.

- *Diet.* Dietary risks include high protein intake, high fat intake, high caffeine intake, and overweight.

The list of breast cancer risk factors is lengthy; most women fit into at least one risk category. The degree to which each risk contributes to the actual development of breast cancer has not been fully assessed. (See the following question for a closer look at dietary risks.)

∗ Can my diet affect my chances of getting breast cancer?

The United States and northern Europe have a breast cancer rate five to six times higher than most Asian or African countries. Some researchers believe that the significant difference in cancer rates has to do with the differences in diet. We eat a large amount of animal protein (milk, meat, eggs, cheese) and fat. In the U.S., breast cancer rates rise proportionately to income. The affluent also have diets rich in protein, cholesterol, and fat. When fed to animals, this diet increased the growth of breast cancers. On the other hand, a low-fat, moderate-protein intake may be protective.

Excessive weight may also promote breast cancer by setting up a metabolic environment that promotes tumor growth. In women who have had breast cancer, the leaner women had the best success with treatment. The highest treatment failure was for women who weighed 170 pounds or more.

To control your dietary risks for breast cancer, lower your fat intake (both animal fats and vegetable oils), eat moderate amounts of protein (no 16-ounce steaks!) and work at maintaining your ideal weight.

MENSTRUAL DISTRESS

* Can herbal teas help menstrual discomfort?

For centuries herbal teas have been recommended to ease discomfort so it's no wonder they are suggested to relieve menstrual cramping and pain. Pennyroyal, mint, camomile, rosemary, and peppermint are all supposed to provide some relief. Remember, a warm beverage, herbal or not, may be soothing to a cramped abdomen. A cup or two of herbal tea might be a comforting change, but keep in mind that herbs have pharmacological (druglike) properties and must be used in moderation. (See the question "I enjoy herbal teas but have been warned they can cause bad reactions. . . ." in Chapter 3.)

* What helps menstrual depression?

Supplementation with vitamin B_6 has successfully relieved premenstrual depression and the depression associated with oral-contraceptive use.

Estrogen-containing oral contraceptives and periods of the month when estrogen levels are high in the body adversely effect the action of B_6. This, in turn, alters brain chemistry and may result in depression. There is considerable evidence to show that a person's mood is affected by concentrations of specific chemicals in certain parts of the brain. Lowered levels are associated with depression. Daily supplements of 10 milligrams of B_6 have successfully relieved these mood swings in some women. Ten milligrams is a large dose since 2 milligrams is the normal daily requirement.

We are not suggesting that B_6 supplementation is a panacea for depressive illness, but if you experience mood cycles, why not try a supplement for three months? It might prove helpful. (See the question "Which vitamin should I take to relieve my feelings of depression?" later in this chapter.)

* Are there any nutritional "cures" for menstrual cramps?

Menstrual cramps are the most common cause of lost working time among women. Some women experience mild discomfort while others are truly incapacitated two days out of every month. The symptoms and severity differ among women and often change month to month. Stress seems to worsen the condition but symptoms can occur during very relaxed times as well. For years, these symptoms—abdominal bloating, weight gain, sore breasts, irritability, depression, fatigue, headache, backache, and joint pain—were ignored by the medical profession. Women who complained were considered neurotic, hysterical, or simply looking for an excuse for a "sick day." The premenstrual syndrome (PMS) is now recognized and treated seriously. Women may experience it shortly before their monthly period or at midcycle. The cyclic body changes and mood swings have even been reported to occur after menopause.

Many authorities suggest diet changes to relieve monthly discomfort. For a week to ten days before your next period, try the following: eating small, frequent, high-protein meals can help the symptoms of irritability, headache, fatigue, and aggression. Try to resist the craving for sweets that often occurs premenstrually. High-carbohydrate and high-salt intakes can contribute to bloating and weight gain. Regular exercise, adequate rest, and little or no alcohol also proves helpful. For breast soreness and swelling cut out coffee, tea, chocolate, and cola drinks. For some this may have to be a consistent elimination rather than for just a short time each month. (For more information see the other questions in this section and the question "Can eliminating coffee reduce my breast lumps?" in the Breast Problem section of this chapter.)

NUTRITION FOR MENOPAUSE

∗ I have seen those commercials on TV that say women need additional iron. Do I still need this after menopause?

You are no longer losing iron monthly through menstrual bleeding so you are less likely to be iron deficient. The RDA for women over fifty-one is 10 milligrams, down from 18 milligrams for premenopausal women.

Although we would not recommend an iron supplement to all women your age, some older women may need supplemental iron and all older women should conscientiously eat good food sources of iron. (See the chart "Iron in Food" in Chapter 2's Mineral Section. Also note the chart "Meeting a Woman's Iron Needs Through Food" earlier in this chapter.) As you can see, even a varied diet just meets your iron needs for the day. And we are presuming optimum absorption of iron. This just is not true all the time. Many things interfere with iron utilization: high intakes of tea and whole grains; chronic conditions such as hemorrhoids and diverticular disease; use of antacids and other drugs; and ill-fitting dentures, which narrow food selection, just to name a few.

Evaluate your normal diet and decide if your daily iron intake is adequate. If you feel you are not getting enough, a supplement of 5 to 10 milligrams a day might be beneficial.

∗ I am menopausal; should I take extra vitamins?

Specific nutritional guidelines for menopause are unknown. Reliable information is unavailable and recommendations suggested are not based on scientific evidence. We would have said in the past that a varied diet, moderate in calories would provide all of your nutritional needs. For older women that simply may not be true.

The RDA for calories for women age fifty-one to seventy-five averages 1,800 calories a day with a range of 1,400 to 2,200 depending on activity and body size. When daily calories fall much below 1,800, it is difficult to select foods that meet your nutritional needs. There are no calories to spare for an occasional drink or dessert. If a frivolous choice replaces a good choice the person's nutrient intake suffers. No one need eat their exact RDA requirement daily but the point is older women need fewer calories and it is easier for them to be short in certain nutrients. Remember, too, that a menopausal woman may have arrived at this point in her life nutritionally drained by numerous pregnancies.

We feel the menopausal woman must consider her nutrient needs carefully. Not only should she eat well, but a vitamin-mineral supplement may be in order too. Nutrients that are particularly important are vitamin D and calcium to prevent osteoporosis; iron to prevent anemia; vitamin E to relieve symptoms of menopause; and vitamin A and C for tissue and bone maintenance. The following might be used as a guideline for supplementation.

Nutrient	Supplement recommendation	Percent of RDA daily requirement
Vitamin A	2,000 I.U. (400 R.E)	50
Vitamin C	60 mg.	100
Vitamin D	100 I.U. (3.75 mcg.)	50
Vitamin E*	8 I.U.	100
Calcium	800 mg.	100
Iron	5–10 mg.	50–100

* To relieve menopausal discomfort 30 to 300 I.U. per day are recommended.

✳ My friend is taking 1,200 I.U. of vitamin E daily to control hot flashes. Is this safe?

The RDA for vitamin E for women is 8 milligrams daily. Your friend is taking a dose that far exceeds this requirement. We'd urge caution when taking such a large daily dose.

Whopping amounts of one nutrient may upset the body's normal balance and may even be toxic. Therapeutic doses, however, may be helpful to correct deficiencies and often are reported to make the user feel better.

Therapeutic doses of vitamin E, 30 to 300 milligrams, have been suggested by some doctors to help minimize severe menopausal symptoms. If a woman experiences hot flashes she might find relief by taking 30 to 300 milligrams of vitamin E daily. The relief she seeks may not be seen for two to six weeks, so the vitamin E intake must be coupled with a dose of patience.

One last note: Vitamin E is a fat soluble vitamin. It is absorbed from the intestinal tract along with fat and in turn aids in the absorption of unsaturated fats. Therefore, a vitamin E supplement will be most thoroughly absorbed if taken at the end of a meal that contains some fat. It is least likely to be absorbed if taken on an empty stomach.

OSTEOPOROSIS AND CALCIUM

* What exactly is osteoporosis?

Osteoporosis is a decrease in bone density without changes in the chemical composition of the bone. The bone is normal but becomes progressively thinner and more fragile. Causes are numerous. Lack of exercise and prolonged low-calcium intakes are very important factors. High meat diets, high phosphorous, low vitamin D intake, numerous pregnancies, and menopause are contributing factors. While thought of as a disease of old age, osteoporosis usually begins decades before your gray hair appears. As early as twenty-five a small percent of Americans show reduced bone density.

Prevention is the best treatment—exercise coupled with adequate calcium, vitamin D, and flouride intakes. (See the box "To Combat Osteoporosis.")

To Combat Osteoporosis

Do	Don't
exercise regularly.	eat excessive amounts of
eat calcium rich foods daily.	meat.
take a daily calcium	drink large amounts of soda.
supplement.	use excessive amounts of
drink fluoridated water.	antacids.
eat adequate sources of	
vitamin D.	

---

* Is osteoporosis an inevitable condition that all women must face because of the decrease in estrogen production that occurs after menopause?

Osteoporosis (thin bones) is a reduction in the quantity of bone in the skeleton, causing the bones to be more fragile. At some point after age thirty-five the bone loss begins. The underlying cause of osteoporosis is not completely understood. One theory is that the decrease of estrogen, common in menopausal and post-menopausal women, may contribute to osteoporosis. This theory gained support when it was observed that women who had hysterectomies in their late twenties and early thirties occasionally developed osteoporosis as early as age forty. Estrogen was suggested as the agent that might counteract the condition and stimulate bone formation. So began estrogen therapy for osteoporosis. However, in the late sixties and early seventies even though estrogen was widely prescribed as an aging preventive, the osteoporosis rate continued to rise.

Currently estrogen therapy to prevent osteoporosis is controversial. A combined treatment with estrogen and calcium supplementation is under investigation as a new way to handle osteoporosis.

Osteoporosis, like menopause, cannot be separated from the aging process. However, many people who show bone loss when X-rayed still remain in vigorous health, without fractures or any discomforts. This continued vigor can usually be attributed to exercise and sensible nutrition. Some authorities feel that calcium supplementation coupled with a good diet and exercise may help to prevent osteoporosis. And the earlier one starts this regimen the better. Read the remaining questions in this chapter for more specific information.

* My mother was five feet three inches until she was fifty-five years old, then she actually shrunk two full inches. Will I?

Most people find that after age fifty they become an inch or more shorter than they used to be. There are several reasons for this. One reason is that the connective tissue disks between the vertebrae of the spine shrink. Also osteoporosis, with its loss of bone tissue, is found mainly in the backbone. These two changes cause the spine to shorten, which reduces height. Additionally, as you grow older (especially females) there is a curvature or "bowing in" of the spine that contributes to height loss. The "bowing in" of the spine also causes the stomach muscles to lose tone so that the belly sticks out.

Some loss of height is unavoidable, but you may be able to minimize it with regular exercise. Stooped posture and rounded shoulders can make you look shorter, so be aware of your posture and remember to stand as straight as possible— as if there were a string hanging from the ceiling attached to the top of your head.

* Why are women more likely to get osteoporosis?

Optimum bone density is reached in women at about age thirty-five. After that the weakening process begins and if no preventive measures are taken one in four post-menopausal women will have osteoporosis. In men, this condition effects only one in eight.

Women are more susceptible to osteoporosis because they start out with bones that are smaller and less dense than men's, in part because women tend to be less active. Pregnancy, breast feeding, and frequent dieting also strain the body's calcium reserves leading to reduced bone density. At menopause, the hormonal changes that occur further accelerate bone loss. And lastly, women live longer than men, which increases their chances of suffering the consequences of a progressive chronic condition.

Lack of exercise, numerous pregnancies, frequent dieting, menopause, and aging may result in a prolonged deficiency of calcium, leading to bone loss with consequent weakening and susceptibility to fracture. A deficiency of as little as 50 milligrams of calcium a day (the amount found in three tablespoons of milk) over a twenty-year period can cause osteoporosis. Estimates suggest that most women consume less than 50 percent of their required calcium each day.

* I read a magazine article that said fluoride supplements can cure osteoporosis. How much should I take?

Treating osteoporosis with fluoride supplements is still experimental but the potential looks very promising. Researchers at Mayo Clinic treated patients with large doses of sodium fluoride combined with calcium. The sodium fluoride appears to stimulate bone formation returning the bone to a normal state. Dr. Riggs, who headed the study, feels we may be able to offer wide-scale fluoride treatment within five years. In the meantime, drinking fluoridated water will offer some protection. Those who have lived most of their lives in high-fluoride areas have a lowered incidence of osteoporosis regardless of their calcium consumption.

* Can vitamin D cure osteoporosis?

The hormone form of vitamin D, calcitriol (Rocaltrol) has been used to treat osteoporosis. It appears to increase absorption of dietary calcium and uptake of calcium by the bone. Normally, conversion to the hormone form of the vitamin occurs through the combined action of the liver and kidneys. As we age, however, our ability to manufacture this hormone declines. Supplementation helps make up for the deficit.

Researchers are looking more closely at the role of vitamin D in the prevention and treatment of osteoporosis. Some have even suggested that the RDA for vitamin D, 200 I.U. (5 micrograms) should be increased to 400 I.U. (10 micrograms) to prevent bone loss as we age.

* Is osteomalacia the same as osteoporosis?

No. Osteoporosis is bone thinning with no change in the mineral composition of the bone. Osteomalacia is bone softening resulting from a loss of bone minerals.

Contrary to popular belief, bones are constantly changing. Minerals, especially calcium, are continually removed and replaced in bones. Occasionally this mineral balance is disrupted. Inadequate amounts of vitamin D cause more calcium to be lost than replaced, resulting in demineralization. Aluminum-containing antacids (Maalox, Amphojel) block bone absorption of phosphates. Prolonged or excessive use can cause the bone damage of osteomalacia.

A recent medical journal report cited just such a case. A sixty-year-old woman suffering from hiatus hernia had been using Maalox for years, when she decided to triple her daily antacid dose. Within six months she was hospitalized for weakness and pain. The diagnosis was osteomalacia due to phosphate malabsorption. An antacid without aluminum was substituted and within a few months her mineral balance returned to normal and her symptoms disappeared.

* I'm fifty-five, how much calcium do I need each day?

Women need more calcium than men to insure the integrity of their bones as they age. Each year 6 million Americans, most of them white, post-menopausal women, suffer bone fractures. This progressive loss and weakening of bones can be slowed by adequate calcium. The RDA for adult women is 800 milligrams. Most authorities recommend greater amounts to slow down bone loss—1,000 to 1,200 milligrams daily. To consume that much calcium would require drinking more than one quart of milk daily, or eating the equivalent amount of calcium in foods such as cheese, greens, and canned salmon.

We feel women need calcium supplements because most likely they will not consume optimum calcium levels through diet alone. We'd recommend a supplement of 800 milligrams a day plus a minimum intake of two glasses of milk plus other calcium-containing foods. The additional food choices should bring your calcium intake within the range suggested for optimum bone health. (See the other questions in this section on osteoporosis as well as the chart "Calcium in Food.")

* I don't drink much milk. Are there other good sources of calcium?

You may not drink milk out of habit, or because you don't like it, or because you are intolerant to it. If habit is the reason, we'd encourage you to try to change. It's to your advantage as a woman to get at least 1 gram (1,000 milligrams) of calcium a day, and milk is an excellent source. Try a small portion—a juice glass—of milk with a meal. Or try an ice cube in milk—some find *very* cold milk refreshing.

If you are intolerant of milk or you simply don't enjoy it there are other good sources of calcium: cheese, green leafy vegetables, and sardines are just a few. (See the chart "Calcium in Foods.")

Keep in mind that you need not drink all your milk. You can eat some as yogurt, custard, cream soup, or as a sauce in a casserole. If you cook with milk use protein-fortified skim milk (like Light n' Lively), since it has more calcium than regular whole or skim milk.

* Is chicken soup a good source of calcium?

We've heard that recommendation before. People suggest chicken soup as a good source of calcium assuming that the

CALCIUM IN FOODS

Food	Portion	Milligrams of calcium
Almonds	12 nuts	38
Beef	3 ounces	10
Bread, white enriched	1 slice	24
Bread, whole-wheat	1 slice	24
Broccoli	½ cup	68
Butter	1 tablespoon	3
Cheese, American	1 ounce (1 slice)	195
Cheese, cheddar	1 ounce	204
Cheese, cottage, creamed	¼ cup	34
Cheese, cream	1 ounce	23
Cheese, mozzarella (whole milk)	1 ounce	163
Cheese, Swiss	1 ounce	259
Collards	1 cup	357
Crackers, graham	2 crackers	10
Custard	½ cup	161
Egg	1 medium	28
Ice cream	½ cup	99
Margarine	1 pat	2
Milk, buttermilk	1 cup	296
Milk, nonfat dry (reconstituted)	1 cup	298
Milk, skim (1% fat)	1 cup	300
Milk, skim plus milk solids (protein fortified)	1 cup	349
Milk, whole	1 cup	291
Nuts, Brazil	4 nuts	28
Oatmeal, cooked	½ cup	11
Orange juice	1 cup	25
Peanuts, roasted without skin	1 tablespoon	5
Peas, cooked	½ cup	22
Perrier water	1 cup	32
Salmon	3 ounces	167
Sardines	3 ounces	372

Food	Portion	Milligrams of calcium
Shrimp	3 ounces	98
Spinach	1 cup	51
Tofu	3 ounces	128
Tuna	3 ounces	7
Tums (antacid)	1 tablet	200
Turkey	3 ounces	7
Walnuts	¼ cup	41
Yogurt	1 cup	293

calcium from the chicken bones leaches into the soup. This doesn't happen since the soup is not acidic enough to soak out the calcium. Even the best homemade chicken soup, though it might relieve a stuffy nose, won't improve the strength of your bones.

Canned chicken soup is also very low in calcium, one bowl (approximately 8 ounces) will provide 3 to 15 milligrams of calcium, depending on the brand and variety (broth, noodle, rice, or vegetable).

* Is dolomite the best calcium supplement?

Although widely used and avidly recommended by magazines and health food stores, we don't recommend dolomite as a calcium supplement. *Dolomite* is a rock composed chiefly of calcium and magnesium, but samples vary and some have been heavily contaminated by toxic minerals like lead, arsenic, mercury, and aluminum.

Physicians have reported unusual symptoms that were eventually traced to excessive dolomite use and probable heavy metal poisoning. A famous case is that of an actress whose health was destroyed by crippling lead poisoning resulting from prolonged dolomite use.

Chemically, dolomite is calcium magnesium carbonate. Proponents claim the magnesium aids the absorption of calcium in the body. This is not true. Pharamacists may add magnesium to calcium supplements to reduce constipation, but it does not aid absorption.

Bone meal, also recommended as a calcium supplement, has been shown to be unrealiable since samples may contain undesirably high levels of lead. We would not recommend its use. (See the following question.)

* Which is the best calcium supplement?

Calcium lactate or calcium carbonate are probably the cheapest sources of nonfood calcium you can find. Calcium gluconate may be used also. Drugstores and supermarkets often have an inexpensive generic brand of one of these that is good to use. Calcium tablets are large, which might make them difficult to swallow. Crushing or breaking the tablet is fine. You might even mix it with a spoonful of food such as cooked cereal or applesauce. There is a misconception that if the tablets are crushed or capsules opened calcium will be absorbed more efficiently. Since calcium is absorbed in varying degrees throughout the small intestine, crushing tablets or opening capsules is of no advantage. Do so only if it helps you to swallow the supplement more easily.

A calcium suspension, a liquid supplement, is available and can be very useful. Calcium carbonate suspension provides 1.6 grams calcium per tablespoon, which meets your daily need. Check with your druggist if you want to use a liquid supplement. One note of caution: Prolonged use of calcium carobonate may cause constipation; however, many of these supplements have magnesium added to relieve this side effect.

We have not recommended dolomite or bone meal as calcium supplements. See the preceding question for our reasons.

* My bottle of calcium recommends six pills a day. Why?

To increase absorbability calcium supplements are made as an organic salt, calcium plus another compound, such as lactate, carbonate, or gluconate. The process makes the pill very bulky. Each tablet may contain 100 to 200 milligrams of calcium. To provide 800 milligrams a day requires taking four to eight tablets. Usually the dose is divided into three times daily. We'd recommend taking each dose with half a glass of milk. The lactose (milk sugar) increases calcium absorption and establishes the habit of drinking milk daily. (See the questions "I'm fifty-five, how much calciuum do I need each day?" and "Which is the best calcium supplement?" in this section.)

* How can eating a diet with large amounts of meat cause my bones to become thin?

A high-protein intake can cause increased calcium loss from the body. When calcium is lost and not adequately replaced, bone thinning (osteoporosis) may result.

High phosphorous intake can also interfere with calcium absorption. High protein foods—meat, fish, poultry—are quite high in phosphorus. The calcium-phosphorus ratio of our diets affects our bones. When phosphorus is consumed in far greater amounts than calcium, the calcium is withdrawn from the bone, causing weakening. The ideal ratio is 1:1. Milk comes close to this with 298 milligrams of calcium and 234 milligrams of phosphorus in a cup. In other foods, the balance is tilted toward phosphorus, resulting in lowered calcium absorption. The following are a few such examples:

Food	Amount	Milligrams of Calcium	Milligrams of Phosphorus	Ratio
Liver, beef	3½ oz.	7	358	1:44
Gatorade	10 oz.	.8	28	1:35
Chicken breast	4 oz.	19	245	1:19
Flounder	3 oz.	23	344	1:16
Coca-Cola	10 oz.	12	64	1:5.3

Carbonated soda and athletic drinks (note Gatorade and Coca-Cola above) may be high in phosphorus. Heavy consumption of either is not advisable for bone health. Phosphate additives—disodium phosphate, calcium phosphate, sodium pyrophosphate—are being used in processed foods, giving still more phosphorus. Some authorities estimate we are eating four times the amount of phosphorus we need, which may have an adverse effect on our bones.

* What does vitamin D have to do with strong bones?

Vitamin D helps to make and maintain bones. It acts as a hormone, regulating calcium and phosphorus levels in the blood and making the minerals available to the bones as needed for growth and repair. When vitamin D is in short supply bone-mineral regulation is seriously affected.

Most foods are naturally low in vitamin D so we rely heavily on vitamin D fortification for our daily requirement of 200 I.U. (5 micrograms). Vitamin D fortified milk is our major source. If a person drinks little milk or is intolerant to it he may not receive enough vitamin D. Cereals and breakfast cakes are also vitamin D fortified, providing 10 to 25 percent of the U.S. RDA per serving.

Vitamin D can be made in the body. It is the "sunshine" vitamin." Ultraviolet rays of the sun convert vitamin D substances in our skin to the active form. This is not the most dependable source, as was once believed. Fog, smog, clothing, clouds, smoke, window glass, and dark skin all filter out ultraviolet rays, reducing the production of vitamin D. Those who work indoors, underground, or at night receive little or no benefit from the sunlight conversion of vitamin D.

INFECTION, HEADACHES, DEPRESSION, AND STRESS

* I was told to drink cranberry juice because I have a bladder infection. Why?

Cranberry juice, in large amounts, acidifies the urine, which helps to control bladder infection caused by ammonia-producing bacteria. You may be discouraged when you hear that you would have to drink six or more glasses daily to have any effect. This would equal more than 960 calories. There are easier ways to acidify the urine: taking vitamin C—4 or more grams daily—or medications such as K-Phos (potassium acid phosphate) and Uracid (dl-Methionine).

* Can recurrent headaches be caused by something I eat?

Apparently a significant number of migraine headaches are related to food. Dr. Frederic Speer, a noted allergist, states that headaches may be the result of a reaction to milk, kola nuts (cola beverages), corn, eggs, peas (peanuts and legumes too), and cinnamon (nutmeg and bay leaf are relatives that also bear watching). Migraine headaches have also been linked to caffeine, alcoholic beverages, aged cheese, seafood, certain meats (especially pork), citrus fruits, fatty fried foods, and some vegetables (especially onions). Caffeine withdrawal can induce severe headaches. If you've recently cut down on coffee or tea, headaches may be troublesome for a week or two.

Some migraine sufferers report more frequent headaches when they take antibiotics. Since antibiotics change the normal bacteria in the intestines, it is possible that digestion and absorption of food is altered. This could cause greater food sensitivity resulting in more frequent headaches.

Other migraine sufferers are sensitive to food additives. Tartrazine (a yellow food color), sodium nitrate (used to preserve meat), and monosodium glutamate (MSG, a flavor enhancer), can all provoke headache in sensitive people. MSG sensitivity is commonly called "Chinese restaurant syndrome" since these foods are high in this additive. Those susceptible to MSG experience headache and a burning sensation in the back of the neck, across the chest, and over the forearms together with tightness across the chest. The symptoms begin within an hour after the meal and can be provoked by as little as one teaspoon of MSG.

If you feel your recurrent headaches may be food related, read the following question.

* How can I tell if my headaches are caused by a food sensitivity?

It's been estimated that roughly 8 percent of the general population suffer from migraines and a certain proportion of these headaches are food related. Many people are unaware of this possible relationship between food and headache, so they continue to eat the food that is causing the problem.

There is some practical advice we can offer migraine sufferers about their diet. A survey of people with recurrent migraines showed that many avoided certain foods because they felt these foods provoked or aggravated attacks. Foods avoided most frequently were chocolate, cheese and dairy foods, citrus fruits, and alcoholic drinks. For a trial period of six weeks, exclude these foods from your diet. You might not realize that your daily cheese sandwich or martini is causing your recurrent headaches. If a headache occurs during the trial period, record all foods eaten twenty-four hours prior to the attack. Note any foods infrequently eaten. In a week or so, challenge yourself with the same amount of this food and see if a headache is provoked.

After the six-week trial is over, during which you've eaten no chocolate, dairy, citrus, or alcoholic food, begin to add back to your diet these common offenders. If headaches return you should be able to tell what food is the problem. (For more information on food allergies, see Chapter 9.)

* Which vitamin should I take to relieve my feelings of depression?

We all go through periods of depression and it's quite normal. Depression can result from excessive dieting, an illness, a life change, or "change of life." If you are suddenly coping with high blood pressure, a new job, the children leaving home, or menopause you may be suffering from mild depression.

Both vitamins and minerals have been recommended as a treatment. Orthomolecular psychiatry is firmly based on the idea that some of our severe mental problems are associated with nutrient imbalances. We are not so sure. We've read the evidence and evaluated it carefully. Our conclusion, at this point, is that we simply do not know enough to make sweeping generalizations about the nutritional treatment of mental problems and depression. We are taking a "wait-and-see" attitude. Therefore, we cannot recommend a specific nutrient or amount that would be helpful except in the case of menstrual depression. (See the question "What helps menstrual depression?" in this chapter.) Taking a daily multivitamin-mineral supplement in amounts close to the RDA may prove helpful, as will eating varied meals at regular times throughout the day. Poor nutrition can accentuate depression, and skipping meals leads to irritability.

* I have a new job and I'm under a great deal of stress. Will stress vitamins help me?

Stress formula supplements usually contain a mixture of B vitamins and C. They are being promoted aggressively as protection against stress. Throughout history man has intuitively realized that a person's state of mind affects his state of health. In recent years, significant research has been done on the connection between illness and stress. The research, however, is often contradictory, making conclusions difficult. As the stress-illness puzzle continues to evolve, nutritionists are attempting to discover how stress alters nutrient requirements.

Blood levels of vitamins do change in response to stress and body potassium levels decrease. Little is known about the body's response to job stress (like meeting deadlines or fighting with a co-worker) since most research has focused on the stress caused by physical trauma or severe illness. Clinical reports show beneficial effects from vitamin C supplementation in stress conditions caused by burns, injuries, sur-

---

STRESS AND YOUR DIET

Do	Don't
eat foods rich in vitamin C.	take stress formula vitamins.
eat nutrient-rich foods.	overeat.
drink fruit juice rich in potassium (orange, tomato).	abuse drugs or alcohol hoping to relax.
exercise regularly.	
take a daily vitamin-mineral supplement.	

gery, and infection. There is no solid evidence that vitamin C supplementation is useful for job-related stress.

Change of job is rated number 19 out of 43 as a life event that produces stress. The stress you are feeling could affect your health. A vitamin-mineral supplement with amounts close to the RDA plus some additional vitamin C may be helpful and at worst will cause no harm. Also, try exercising to relieve muscular tension. Eat well but do not overeat, since stress slows down the production of digestive enzymes and this can lead to indigestion. (See the highlight box "Stress and Your Diet" for further hints.)

6

Trouble With Indigestion?

All through recorded history, mankind has been concerned with digestion and its upsets. The Egyptians thought that most illness originated in the intestinal tract. They made a habit of fasting and took drugs that caused vomiting at regular intervals.

Peppermint, antimony, raw garlic, gold mixtures, coffee, and hot chocolate have been used to treat indigestion throughout the ages. The famous French gourmet Brillat-Savarin recommended "a good size cup of fine chocolate" after a heavy lunch to ensure complete digestion within three hours. Some of these aids probably aggravated the condition because we know now that peppermint, coffee, and chocolate may actually cause heartburn.

Most of us are bothered with discomforts of indigestion at one time or another and maybe more frequently than that. Nausea, heartburn, belching, stomachache, gas, sour taste in the mouth, cramps, constipation, and diarrhea, are, unfortunately, familiar to us all. We spend over $450 million each year on antacids and more than one-fourth of middle-age Americans (forty-five and over) take laxatives more than three times a week.

We feel good nutrition coupled with positive health habits could reduce our reliance on laxatives and antacids. The highlight boxes in the chapter will help you gain relief from discomfort.

139

✳ What can I do to reduce indigestion?

First, you should see a physician to rule out any physical cause for your indigestion. In most cases, indigestion is due to irrational tension or to an intolerance to certain food.

Some foods and drinks are known to increase the production of stomach acid—alcohol, coffee, tea, cola, pepper, chili powder, and foods high in protein. Eliminate or reduce your use of these spices and beverages. When you eat foods high in protein, eat them along with other foods to reduce their concentration. Fats reduce acid secretion.

Bland diets (those that do not contain fried food, dried peas or beans, fibrous fruits or vegetables, or spices) have been suggested for indigestion. Many of these excluded foods have not been shown to irritate the stomach. It is probably best to note which specific foods *you* don't tolerate well and omit these.

How often and *where* you eat may be as important or even more important than *what* you eat. Be sure to eat three small meals regularly supplemented by two snacks. Never overeat. Snacktimes should be mid-morning and mid-afternoon, never at bedtime. Take your meals and snacks in a pleasant, peaceful environment when possible, and eat slowly and calmly.

ANTACIDS

✳ I take antacids for indigestion because my stomach is too acid. My neighbor said I could use milk instead. Is that true?

Many people complain of indigestion—pain, burning, belching, bloating, regurgitation of food into the mouth, nausea, and gas. But rest assured these unpleasant signs are not because of acid in your stomach. Your stomach has to be acid to do its job. Normal stomach acidity, measured as pH, is 2.0. (You can compare that with the pH of vinegar, which is 2.9; the lower the pH the stronger the acid.) So you see there really is nothing to the "acid indigestion" they speak about in the ads for antacids. Too much or too little does not cause indigestion.

People have been using milk for years to relieve the discomfort of indigestion. It isn't very good for that, for a few reasons. First of all, because it is a liquid, it leaves the stomach fast; second, milk itself stimulates acid secretion in the stomach; and third, while milk can neutralize (buffer) the acid, it has a limited capacity to do this compared with antacids.

While antacids do what their name implies—neutralize acids—there are some problems that may develop when using them for a long time. (See the following question.)

Why not try a few changes in what you eat and how you eat to see if you can reduce your indigestion without resorting to antacids. (See the highlight box "Bothered with Indigestion?")

* Can long-term use of antacids be a problem?

There are over eight thousand different brands of antacids available. These are used to neutralize (buffer) stomach acid. Because of this, they all interfere with iron absorption and may cause a deficiency. Don't take an iron supplement with an antacid, separate the doses by at least two to three hours. Most usually contain calcium carbonate (Tums), aluminum hydroxide and magnesium oxide (Di-Gel, Maalox, Mylanta), aluminum hydroxide and magnesium trisilicate (Gelusil), magnesium hydroxide (milk of magnesia), and sodium bicarbonate (Alka-Seltzer). All these, except for milk of magnesia, also contain sodium.

Excessive use of calcium carbonate causes nausea and constipation. When taken with milk, there is an increase in urinary excretion of calcium that can result in kidney stones. Studies show that several hours after persons take calcium carbonate antacids, they develop high stomach acidity as a rebound response.

Aluminum hydroxide antacids, if overused, block phosphorus absorption and calcium is lost in the urine as the kidneys try to balance the minerals in the blood. Long-term use can contribute to bone disorders like osteomalacia and osteoporosis. (See Chapter 5 for more about this.) They also cause constipation.

Magnesium-containing antacids are very effective, but prolonged use will cause diarrhea. That is why the most often used antacids combine aluminum and magnesium. That way the bowels may be unaffected.

Sodium bicarbonate—containing antacids, unlike most other antacids, are absorbed and can cause problems if taken too often. If you are on a low-sodium diet, you should never use sodium bicarbonate antacids. Alka-Seltzer contains 276 milligrams of sodium in one tablet. A list of the sodium content of commonly used antacids is in Chapter 8.

Antacids should be taken only if needed and taken for extended periods only under the direction of a physician. They should be taken one to three hours after meals. An additional dose is usually given at bedtimes. (See the question "Which is the best antacid to use?" in Chapter 4.)

BOTHERED WITH INDIGESTION?

Do	*Don't*
eat slowly and calmly.	overeat.
eat in a pleasant place.	snack at bedtime.
eat three small meals plus two snacks.	drink coffee, tea, alcohol, or cola.
eat some fat at each meal or snack.	eat pepper or chili powder.

HEARTBURN

* What can I do to avoid heartburn?

Heartburn, a burning sensation felt in the area of the throat and heart has nothing to do with the heart. It is caused by a reflux of food and acid from the stomach into the esophagus (the tube that carries food from the mouth to the stomach). The backing up of stomach contents irritates the esophagus, causing a burning sensation. Sometimes the food and acid pass all the way up to the mouth.

One reason for this backup of food is the strong muscular reaction of the stomach to being stuffed with too much food. A relaxed lower esophageal sphincter (LES) also allows the stomach contents to splash back. A sphincter is a muscle surrounding and closing an opening. In this case, the LES is around the opening between the esophagus and the stomach.

Regular and decaffeinated coffee, chocolate, alcohol, food high in fat, and the flavorings peppermint and spearmint all relax the LES (we guess crème de menthe does not deserve its reputation as a digestive aid). Cigarette smoking relaxes the muscle too. If you wish to prevent heartburn, you should avoid these foods, drinks, and cigarettes. (Skim milk increases LES pressure so it may be helpful.)

Overweight, especially extra fat on the belly and the pressure it causes on the abdomen, increases the chance of food refluxing back. You will have an easier time avoiding heartburn if your weight is normal. Lying down, lifting something heavy, and even bending over can start the backing up process that results in heartburn.

This response is exaggerated by eating a large meal, so it is best to eat smaller amounts more often—three small meals a day with a mid-afternoon and mid-morning snack. Avoid any food in the last two hours before you go to bed. Keep

---

BOTHERED WITH HEARTBURN?

Do	Don't
reduce if overweight.	stuff yourself.
drink skim milk.	drink coffee (regular or decaffeinated).
eat smaller meals.	drink alcohol.
eat a mid-morning and mid-afternoon snack.	eat chocolate, foods rich in fat, peppermint, or spearmint.
drink liquids in between meals.	smoke cigarettes.
	lie down right after eating.
	exercise after eating.
	eat in the last two hours before bedtime.

away from liquids for one hour before and after each meal or snack. Drink liquids in between mealtimes.

Because heartburn may be a symptom of hiatus hernia, see the next question. Also see the question "Will switching to decaffeinated coffee relieve my heartburn?" in Chapter 4's Caffeine section.

✳ My sister has a hiatus hernia. What foods should she avoid?

More women than men have hiatus hernias—where the stomach slides through the esophageal opening and into the chest cavity. In other words, part of the stomach protrudes through the diaphragm. Causes can be obesity, pregnancy, severe coughing, wearing clothes that are tight around the waist, and even weight lifting. Is is estimated that half of all adults in this country have a mild degree of hiatus hernia, but only a few have symptoms.

There are several things your sister can do to relieve the major symptoms—heartburn, pressure in the abdomen, and more rarely, the feeling of food sticking in the throat. Losing weight is most important. A low-fat diet that is high in protein will help maintain pressure in the lower esophageal sphincter, LES (for an explanation see preceding question). This pressure will keep the sphincter closed and the food in the stomach where it belongs after it is swallowed.

She should eat smaller amounts of food several times a day instead of three large meals. It is particularly important that the evening meal be small. If she usually is uncomfortable after she's in bed, it is better not to eat any more food after dinner. (That may help her to lose weight too.)

Bland foods have been recommended for periods when there is discomfort. But there are many misconceptions about which foods are bland. Many spices and highly seasoned "hot" foods are nonirritating. Black pepper, chili powder, coffee, cocoa, tea, and alcohol are irritants and should be avoided. Fiber or roughage is usually restricted, although there is no agreement that it's irritating. Because constipation and straining to pass stools increases pressure within the abdomen, it's good to eat enough fiber to prevent constipation.

Antacids usually are taken one hour after meals and at

bedtime. They neutralize (buffer) the hydrochloric acid of the stomach and raise the pressure of the lower esophageal sphincter (LES).

Lying down or exercise after meals can cause discomfort. Placing a wedge between the spring and mattress so that the head of the bed is raised four to ten inches higher than the foot will make her more comfortable. Sleeping on a couple of pillows is a simple substitute for this when away from home. Clothes that are tight around the waist and midriff also cause discomfort.

GAS

* I must be a gas producer. I often have rumbling and distention. What foods cause gas?

We are all gas producers—some of us produce more, others less. If you are fortunate and expel it as soon as it is produced, you won't have the same bloating and discomfort as when the gas builds up in the intestine.

Some of the gas, about 70 percent, is swallowed air. Everyone swallows some air when they eat or drink. It may be that some nervous people or people who breathe through their mouth swallow more than the usual amount. Eating slowly with your mouth closed and drinking slowly, instead of gulping, will reduce the amount of air swallowed. Drinkng through a straw rather than gulping from a cup will also help. Chewing gum also leads to swallowed air. This swallowed air plus gas produced from the bacteria fermenting undigested foods in the intestine is what is making you uncomfortable.

Some foods, like beans, have a reputation for being gas producers. The reputation is well deserved. Different kinds of beans produce varying amounts of gas. Other foods such as onions, celery, carrots, raisins, broccoli, cabbage, cauliflower, bananas, apricots, prune juice, pretzels, bagels, cucumbers, radishes, wheat germ, and Brussels sprouts also promote gas formation in some people. Surprisingly, applesauce promotes gas too. Carbonated sodas contain a lot of carbon dioxide that causes belching as it adds to the gas in your body.

Some people are unable to digest lactose, the sugar in milk, and they may suffer from gas produced as bacteria ferment the undigested sugar. (For more about this, see the question "I was told that I have lactose intolerance. . . ." in this chapter.)

If you have recently begun to add more fiber to your diet, you may find that you have more gas than usual. You may adjust to the extra fiber in time. It usually takes about three weeks.

It is helpful to keep a diary and record everything you eat and your gassy episodes. Then you will be able to see a connection between specific foods and gas production. It should be a simple matter to eliminate or reduce the quantities you eat of those foods that are the culprits.

* Is there any way to cook beans so they are less likely to cause gas?

Beans contain some natural sugars that are difficult to digest and so they ferment in the intestine, causing gas. Soak the beans for three hours and discard the soaking water. Cover the beans with fresh water and cook thirty minutes. Once again, drain off the water, rinse the beans thoroughly, cover them with fresh water, and cook until tender. This method should result in less gassy beans.

BOTHERED WITH GAS?

<u>Do</u>	<u>Don't</u>
keep a record of what you eat and when you become gassy.	eat foods with a high gas content, such as whipped cream and soda.
reduce fat in your meals.	talk while chewing, as it will make you swallow more air.
walk after eating rather than lying down.	drink large amounts of milk if you can't digest lactose.
	eat the gas-producing foods.

LACTOSE INTOLERANCE

* What is lactose intolerance?

Lactose is the sugar in milk, both skim and regular. Many of us, after early childhood, are not able to digest this sugar. Africans, Greeks, and Orientals are more likely to have this problem, called "lactose intolerance," than are people of north European ancestry, but many adults of all ethnic groups have it.

People with this disorder develop gas, diarrhea, cramps, and bloating after they drink milk or eat any foods containing milk. This is because the undigested milk acts like a laxative and ferments to produce gas. Some find that they can use small amounts of milk, less than one cup, without ill effects. If the milk is drunk with meals, it is easier to tolerate. Chocolate milk may be used in place of unflavored milk, as it is less likely to cause a reaction.

Most cheeses contain little of the lactose in milk so they are good substitutes. Yogurt has had most of its lactose changed to lactic acid (that's the tangy taste) as has sour cream and cultured buttermilk. They may be eaten with no discomfort.

* I was told that I have lactose intolerance. Can I drink any milk at all?

Many people with lactose intolerance can drink small amounts of milk, one-half cup or so. Take it at mealtimes, along with other food. For some, chocolate milk is tolerated better, maybe because the chocolate slows down digestion.

If you get symptoms of gas, diarrhea, and cramping from even small amounts of milk, you should try the product Lact-Aid.* This is an enzyme preparation that acts on the sugar in milk and changes it to a form you can digest. You can buy this product in the drugstore. You put a few drops of Lact-Aid into

---

* The product can be ordered by mail from SugarLo Company, P. O. Box 111, 600 Fire Road, Pleasantville, New Jersey, 08232; toll-free telephone number: (800) 257-8650.

milk the night before you will use it. By the morning the milk will have little lactose left and you can enjoy it without any discomfort. In some areas of the country Lact-Aid fluid milk is available in the dairy case in the supermarket.

LAXATIVES AND CONSTIPATION

   * My husband said that I am poisoning my body because I don't have a daily bowel movement. Should I take a laxative?

   Many of us were taught that if we didn't move our bowels every day, toxins would build up and poison our bodies. There's no truth in that; it's an old wives' tale. You really don't need a daily bowel movement for good health. Some healthy people defecate every other day or even every third day, while others have movements two or three times a day. It really doesn't matter. You are not necessarily constipated if you don't defecate daily. Constipation refers to the infrequent, and maybe difficult, passage of dry, hard stools.

   If you comfortably pass normally formed movements at regular intervals, there is certainly no need for a laxative.

   * I have gotten into the habit of taking a laxative every night. What can I do to become "regular" without using laxatives?

   First of all you should stop using the laxative completely. That way you help your colon become independent from laxative stimulation. It won't hurt you if you don't have a movement for a day or two. Plan a time every day for a bowel movement. It's a good idea to make this some time soon after breakfast because eating stimulates the response to defecate. Some people find the old practice of drinking a glass of warm water and lemon juice when they first wake up is sufficient stimulus for a bowel movement before breakfast. Allow ten to fifteen minutes on the toilet. Be sure you are seated comfortably. Reading the morning paper is a good way to pass the time and take your mind off straining to hurry the process. Continue this every day, even if you feel you are wasting your time because you do not have an urge. (If you have an urge any other time, heed it.) Think of it like an exercise that will, in time, produce change.

Eat a hearty breakfast, including foods high in fiber such as whole-grain cereals or breads (bran muffins are good; see Chapter 1, Fiber, for recipes). Eat more fiber throughout the day (see Chapter 1 for suggestions). You can use some un-processed bran if you like, but don't overdo it—no more than two or three tablespoons a day with plenty of liquids. A wad of dry bran can itself cause an impaction and interfere with normal movements.

Drink lots of fluids, at least six glasses a day. A glass of prune juice, which has a natural laxative effect, can be part of this. Exercise is important too. A brisk walk before breakfast can stimulate the urge to defecate. Some people have weak stomach wall muscles; one way to strengthen them is by con-tracting the abdomen. Sit-ups and leg lifts also help. (An ex-ercise manual will help you to do these correctly.)

As you substitute the good health habits outlined above for the laxative habit, you will soon have normal, regular bowel movements.

* Is a stool softener like Colace considered a laxative?

Yes, the stool softener Colace is a laxative along with other medications like saline laxatives, lubricants, irritants, and bulk producers, which help to empty the bowels. Each of these types functions in a different way but the end result is the same—they counteract constipation.

Stool softeners like Colace, Disonate, and Surfak increase water retention; in that way they soften the stool.

Lubricants, such as mineral oil, oil the lining of the intes-tine and soften the stool. Because fat soluble vitamins A, D, E, and K dissolve in the mineral oil, they are then carried out of and lost to the body. Habitual use of these lubricants can, after a long while, cause a vitamin deficiency.

Saline laxatives like Epsom Salts, Milk of Magnesia, Sal Hepatica, and Fleet Phospho-Soda, hold and draw water into the intestines. As this water passes out with the feces, it is vital that you drink enough water to replace it. Minerals are also lost this way, and need replacement.

Irritant laxatives like Dulcolax, magnesium citrate, Feen-a-Mint, Senokot, and Cascara Sagrada stimulate movement in the intestine. They frequently cause cramping.

Bulk producers like Metamucil, Cologel, and Hydrolase hold water in the stool and swell up, which aids in the passing of the movement.

All of these laxatives should be used for only a short while. Extended use can cause dependency on them and also loss of water, minerals, and vitamins.

Fiber

✻ I have been constipated since I have been taking an antacid (Amphojel). What can I do to relieve this?

Many medications cause constipation or delay in passing stools. Why not try increasing the amount of fiber you eat everyday? Fiber is very important to normal bowel movements. Indigestible fiber in the intestine absorbs water which softens and increases the size of the stool so that it is passed along the colon faster and excreted more easily. The 1½ grams of fiber you get from two graham crackers can add

---

BOTHERED WITH CONSTIPATION?

Do
establish a pattern of eating
 and elimination.
eat breakfast.
drink a hot beverage first
 thing in the morning.
eat more fiber.
eat prunes and drink prune
 juice for its natural laxative
 effect.
drink six to eight glasses of
 fluid each day.
exercise regularly.

Don't
ignore the urge to defecate.
rush your time in the toilet.
depend on a daily laxative.

PUT A LITTLE FIBER (BULK) IN YOUR LIFE

Step 1: *Eat whole-grain breads and cereals.*
For the first few days eat one serving of whole-grain breads, cereal, pasta, or brown rice. Gradually increase to four or more servings daily.

Step 2: *Eat fresh fruits and vegetables.*
Begin by eating one serving a day of a raw, unpeeled fruit or cooked vegetables including skins. Gradually increase to four servings a day.

Step 3: *Eat dried peas and beans.*
Begin by eating one serving a week (split pea soup, lentils, baked beans, peanuts) and let your taste be your guide. We'd suggest at least two to three servings a week.

Step 4: *Eat unprocessed bran.*
Add bran to your food—cereal, soup, casseroles, muffins (see recipes in Fiber section of Chapter 1) pancakes, baked goods. Start with one teaspoon a day and over a three-week period gradually work up to two to three tablespoons daily. Remember, large amounts of bran are not needed; and drink plenty of liquids along with bran.

---

five to ten times its weight in water to your stool. Fiber also may increase the growth of bacteria that produce fatty acids, which stimulate bowel movements.

Gradually add whole-grain breads and cereals to your meals; increase the amount of fruits and vegetables you eat. Whenever possible, eat them with the peel. You could add small amounts of unprocessed bran—one teaspoon at first—to your food each day. Don't use too much bran, it can cause digestive upset. Two to three tablespoons daily should be your limit. (For other suggestions about fiber, see several questions in Chapter 1's Fiber section and the highlight box "Put a Little Fiber in Your Life," the charts "Foods High in Fiber" and "High Fiber Menus" in this section.)

Along with the extra fiber, be sure to drink plenty of liquids and take a long walk or do some other form of exercise daily.

* Why is prune juice always suggested when you are constipated?

Prune juice is not high in fiber. It helps eliminate constipation because it naturally contains a laxative, dihydroxyphenylisatin. For a morning bowel movement, drink 6 to 8 ounces of prune juice before bedtime. An evening bowel movement can be encouraged by drinking prune juice at breakfast. Prune juice should not be taken each day simply to guarantee a bowel movement. It is high in calories (an 8-ounce glass is 184 calories).

A healthier way to insure regular bowel movements is to eat foods containing fiber, drink lots of liquids, and get regular exercise. See the highlight box "Bothered with Constipation."

FOODS HIGH IN FIBER

Bran	Baked beans
Bran buds and flakes	Peas
Wheat germ	Winter squash
Whole-wheat bread	Broccoli
Peanuts	Apple, with skin
Peanut butter	Pear, with skin
Nuts, all varieties	Strawberries
Sunflower seeds	Blueberries
Dried beans, all varieties	

---

* Which cereals are whole grain?

More and more whole-grain cereals are appearing on the supermarket shelf. Some commonly available varieties are:

Oatmeal	Grape-Nuts
Wheatena	Grape-Nuts Flakes
Ralston	Shredded Wheat
Kasha (buckwheat groats)	Wheaties
Cracked wheat	Crispy Wheats 'n Raisins
Nutri-Grain	Buc Wheats
Granola	

Many other cereals are made of whole grains. Read the labels carefully. Look for the following terms as the first ingredient listed: whole kernel corn, rye, barley, whole wheat, buckwheat, or rolled oats. Be aware that cereals listing as their first ingredient wheat flour, degermed cornmeal, and milled rice are not mainly whole-grain cereals.

HIGH FIBER MENUS

FIRST DAY
Breakfast
Grapefruit (½ or sections)
Oatmeal with milk and raisins
  (add bran if desired)
Bran muffin

Lunch
Cabbage slaw
Tuna salad sandwich with
  celery on whole-wheat bread
Fresh pear with skin

Dinner
Vegetable soup

Broiled fish with sliced almond
  topping
Baked potato with skin
Carrots and peas
Canned crushed pineapple

Snack
Dried fruit and nut mix

SECOND DAY
Breakfast
Orange slices
Grape-Nuts with milk (add bran
  if desired)
Poached egg on whole-wheat
  toast

Lunch
Bean soup
Chef salad (turkey, lettuce,
  tomato, carrot, pepper)
Whole-wheat crackers
Banana

Dinner
Whole-wheat spaghetti with
  meat sauce
Lettuce wedge

Whole-wheat breadsticks
Baked apple

Snack
Graham crackers

HEALTH HINTS

* What should you eat after you have vomited?

Nothing at all for at least one hour. Just lie down quietly and give your digestive tract a chance to rest. Vomiting is the body's way of ridding itself of something irritating. It can result from too much coffee or alcohol, an infection, or food poisoning. The result is the same. You're left weak, mildly dehydrated, and low in some vital body elements—sodium, magnesium, and chloride. You may have an afterbout of severe abdominal gas, which will pass with time.

After the hour is up and you have not vomited again, try a little water—a few sips every few minutes. If that stays down, slowly, and we mean slowly, add other fluids, dry crackers, toast, and cereal. For the next twenty-four hours eat simple carbohydrate foods, drink fluids (ginger ale, cola, grape juice, and weak tea are good) and rest. Bananas, applesauce, and cooked rice or pasta are also good choices. Don't drink milk; it might cause gas and diarrhea in an already irritated stomach.

* Should you "starve a fever and feed a cold" or is it the other way around?

Starving a fever has been practiced for centuries; in some cases even water was withheld. When a person is sick with a fever and infection (cold) he needs liquids and calories to mobilize body defenses to get well.

A feverish person needs plenty of liquid, as much as ten cups and more a day, along with extra calories and protein. In cases of high fever there may be a build-up of gas. This causes an awful bellyache that may be relieved by restricting carbohydrate foods (bread, cereals, etc.), milk, and fat. While the pain persists, if the person is interested in eating at all, he should have only fruit juices and high-protein foods such as eggs, meat, or low-fat cheeses.

* Should you eat when you have diarrhea?

Routinely, people are advised "nothing by mouth" during a bout of diarrhea. Although a traditional practice, there is no real rationale for it since the length of time the diarrhea lasts has no bearing on whether you eat or not. We recommend eating to replace lost fluid, calories, and nutrients.

Go slowly, however. Since your digestive tract is already in turmoil, do not add any more fuel to the fire. If you've had a good bout of diarrhea, you're probably not too hungry. That's okay—just rest. There's no harm if you go without food for six to twelve hours. Simply sip water or suck in ice chips or a Popsicle. You need ten to twelve cups of liquid a day to replace losses, so make sure to take at least one-quarter cup (four tablespoons) every fifteen minutes.

Over the next seventy-two hours, whether the diarrhea continues or not, begin with clear fluids (soda, juice, tea); then full fluids (cream soup, Jell-O); next simple soft foods (cooked cereal, pasta, applesauce), and finally regular meals. When diarrhea is persistent you may not be able to take regular meals, but remember to take whatever you can comfortably. Gatorade, an electrolyte replacement beverage, is sometimes recommended. It's fine, but mix it one to one with water. Taken straight it can aggravate the diarrhea rather than help it. Also stay away from milk, herbal teas, bouillon, butterfat, and foods containing soybeans. Milk can be used only after the diarrhea has been gone for at least twenty-four hours. Occasionally, you will be "milk intolerant" for a few weeks. If, after you drink your first glass of milk, you experience gas and loose stools, you are temporarily intolerant. Simply limit milk (yogurt and cheese should not give you discomfort), and try milk again in two to three weeks, at which point everything should be fine.

7

Slimming Down and Shaping Up the Healthy Way

Almost everyone is a weight watcher these days—trying out or, at the very least, discussing every new diet they read about or hear about. Unfortunately, many of us, weight watchers that we are, are watching our weight go up as the years pass. We'd prefer watching our weight go down or even just remain the same. The average American woman is five feet three inches tall and weighs 143 pounds while the average man is five feet nine inches and weighs 172. Men generally reach their maximum weight and stay there sometime in their mid-forties, women keep gaining until they are in their sixties and then level off.

Something is amiss. Low fat, high fat, low protein, high protein, low carbohydrate, and high carbohydrate, even counting calories—all these diet schemes don't seem to be working very well. At best, they cause a temporary loss of pounds that is almost always regained after a few months. No more than 5 percent of people who lose weight keep it off.

Obviously it's a hard job to retain or regain the slim body you had in your twenties (some of us never had that slim body even then). Is it worth the effort? Recent data suggest that many of us may be aiming for a level of thinness that is neither necessary nor desirable for health and long life. The guide we use here for optimum weight comes from the Metropolitan Life Insurance Height-Weight Table (see Appendix F) which you probably have seen. This table groups into three body types—small, medium, and large. How you decide your body frame is never described. That leaves it subject to your own estimation and this may be colored by your weight: For instance, if your weight fits into the large-frame category, you may decide that you must really have a large frame when it really isn't. (That's a quick way to reach your desirable weight!) It's difficult to judge your body frame size just by looking.

Don't worry about your body frame size too much, as this height-weight table is being revised. The new range of weights will be higher than in the table now. One reason for the revision is that it has been found that good health and long life are to be found within a wide range of weights, up to 20 or 25 percent higher than has been believed best. With this in mind, you may not feel it is worthwhile to try to be much thinner than you are now. In other words, you need not feel guilty if you are carrying ten or so extra pounds. In fact, this is less harmful for your body than losing and gaining ten pounds over and over again.

You may, however, feel you would be more comfortable weighing less. Or you may have high blood pressure, other cardiovascular disease, diabetes, arthritis, or some other disorder that would be helped if you lost some weight. We have some suggestions for you that may help. We have used these with success with people like yourself, who need or want to lose some weight. Why not try these for a month or so and see what happens. We believe you will find your weight going down slowly while you may not even feel that you are "dieting." What you are aiming for is a lifelong change in patterns of food intake.

SUGGESTIONS FOR HOW TO EAT

1. Eat only when you are hungry. This may sound obvious, but think about it for a while, in fact, think about it every time you feel like eating. When you feel like eating, decide if you are really hungry or not. If you are, wait ten minutes before you get something to eat. Don't eat simply because the clock tells you it's time for a meal.

2. Stop eating when you can still eat a little more. (If you wish to linger at the table, have a cup of tea or a glass of club soda or mineral water, all of which are calorie-free, and sip it slowly.)

3. When you are home, eat at one place only. Pick out your favorite seat at the dining-room or kitchen table and sit there every time you eat, even if you are only eating an apple. *Never eat when you are standing.*

4. Eat as slowly as you can. A meal should take at least twenty minutes; a snack ten minutes. Your brain needs time to receive the message that you have eaten. Chew slowly and think about how the food tastes. It helps to put your fork or spoon down between bites instead of using it like a shovel.

5. Don't read or watch TV when eating. Concentrate on eating and on conversation when you eat with someone else.

6. Use a smaller size plate (salad or luncheon plate), so that usual portions of food appear generous.

7. Don't leave snack food around in inviting dishes throughout your home. Keep all foods in one room out of sight in cupboards or in the refrigerator when you are not eating.

8. Practice leaving a little food on your plate. You really don't have to eat it all, even if that's your usual style.

9. Always eat three meals a day. Don't skip a meal because you want to "splurge" later; just eat a little less. Never skip breakfast.

SUGGESTIONS FOR WHAT TO EAT

1. Eat whole-grain breads and cereals and brown rice. They have fewer calories than white bread and refined cereals and are more filling. If you are very hungry before a meal, eat a slice of whole-wheat bread with a glass of water twenty minutes before you eat to take the edge off your appetite.

2. Eat oranges, grapefruit, tomatoes, apples, prunes, and other fruits and vegetables instead of *drinking* their juices.

3. If you must use a spread on bread, use a half teaspoon of jelly or honey for a slice of bread (yes, you can spread it thin enough to cover the slice).

4. Reduce the amount of butter, margarine, or sour cream you use on mashed or baked potatoes. (Use one-half pat of butter, or a smaller dollop of sour cream.) When you have gravy, use less of it. The same goes for salad dressing. If you don't feel ready to substitute a squeeze of lemon or plain vinegar for usual salad dressing, use less of the dressing. Use a tablespoon to measure gravy or salad dressing rather than a ladle or pouring directly from the bottle. Try the Zero Dressing recipe at the end of Chapter 8. You can add salt to it if you want to make it taste more like a usual dressing.

   5. Choose foods that require a lot of chewing—apples, shredded wheat, raw vegetables, dried fruits—because they not only slow down eating, the chewing itself is satisfying.

   6. Eat foods that require effort and slow down eating— nuts and seeds in the shell, unpeeled shrimp, artichokes, half melons.

   7. Avoid fried foods because they are very high in calories. Eat baked, broiled, poached, and steamed foods.

CALORIE COUNTING

* Do I have to count calories if I want to lose weight?

   It has been shown over and over that your weight is simply a reflection of the energy balance in your body. If you take in more calories (energy) than you use, the excess is stored as fat. It's as simple as that. Another thing that has been shown time and again is that knowing the calorie counts of all the food you eat and even totaling them daily does not ensure weight loss.

   Rather than carefully counting out a low-calorie diet, we would rather that you establish positive changes in the way you eat and the food choices you make. Understanding the caloric density of foods is important. It will help you make choices that moderate your calorie intake without the tedious, time-consuming chore of calorie counting.

   A calorie is a measurement of the energy in food. *Calorie density* refers to the number of calories in a portion of food. Some foods have many more calories than others but these are not always the ones you think of as "fattening." Foods that contain a lot of fat have more calories, while foods that contain more carbohydrate or protein have less. This is because weight for weight fat has more than twice as many calories as carbohydrate or protein. This may come as a surprise to you if you have always thought of carbohydrate foods such as bread, potatoes, and rice as being fattening. They really are not when compared to foods high in fat like cheese and nuts.

When you choose food, concentrate on those that are lowest in fat, because these usually will be lowest in calories. If you also choose foods that contain a lot of water and fiber, you will be eating bulky, filling food that has few calories.

Here are a few examples of substitutes you might enjoy.

Avoid	*Use*
French fries	Baked potato
Mashed potatoes	Boiled potato
Candied yams	Baked yams
Creamed corn	Steamed corn
Batter-dipped zucchini	Steamed zucchini
Creamed spinach	Spinach salad
Green beans almondine	Steamed green beans
Tomato juice	Whole tomato
Apple pie	Baked apple
Canned sweetened peaches	Peach in juice (light pack)
Danish pastry	Raisin bread
French toast	Cinnamon toast
Iced chocolate cake	Pound cake
Southern fried chicken	Broiled chicken
Batter-dipped fish	Baked fish
Salisbury steak	Broiled hamburger
Bacon	Canadian bacon
Bologna	Turkey roll
Scrambled egg	Poached egg
Whole milk	Skim milk
Cream cheese	Farmer/low-fat cottage cheese
Ice cream	Frozen yogurt
Cream soup	Clear soup (consommé, broth)

* How many calories a day should I have when I am trying to lose weight?

That depends on how much you weigh at the start. Whenever you take in fewer calories than you need to keep your body going, you withdraw the additional calories from your reserves—body fat. This reduction in body fat leads to a loss in weight. One pound of body fat equals about 3,500 Calories; when, over a period of time, you eat 3,500 Calories less than you use, you will lose one pound. A safe way to do this is by eating 500 to 1,000 Calories less than you need each day. That way you will lose one to two pounds in a week. This doesn't seem like a lot, but if you stick to it, it quickly adds up. And weight that is lost slowly is more apt to stay off.

A quick way to estimate the calories you need each day is to multiply your weight by 14 Calories. If you weigh 140 pounds you need 1,960 Calories each day to maintain your weight. The 14-Calorie-per-pound estimate is for a person who is not very active. If you are active you may need 16 calories or more per pound.

When you have determined how many calories you need each day, you can subtract 500 or 1,000 from that to find the calories you can eat and still lose a pound or two a week. If you weigh 140 pounds, you will lose weight if you eat 1,500 Calories a day.

It is better not to reduce calories below 1,200 a day, or you will be eating too little to get all the nutrients you need and you will feel hungry and deprived and more likely to "cheat."

As men weigh more than women, calorie levels frequently used are 1,600 Calories for men and 1,200 Calories for women. Use these only as a guide. You should be eating enough to allow a small but consistent weight loss.

Your scale may not show that loss exactly. Most bathroom scales are not very accurate and also your weight normally fluctuates apart from what you eat. These fluctuations happen because of water retention or even because you have not had a bowel movement that day.

Don't be too concerned with what you lose each week. Just stick to your new eating habits and you'll reach your goal.

HOW TO ESTIMATE YOUR DESIRABLE WEIGHT

Women	*Men*
100 pounds for first five feet of height, add 5 pounds for each additional inch	106 pounds for first five feet of height, add 6 pounds for each additional inch
5 feet 4 inches	5 feet 9 inches
100 pounds (5 feet)	106 pounds (5 feet)
+ 20 pounds (4 inches)	+ 54 pounds (9 inches)
120 pounds desirable weight	160 pounds desirable weight

* Subtract 5 pounds for each inch less than 5 feet

---

* Will a 600-Calorie diet make me lose weight faster?

In theory, yes, because you would be using up your fat stores more quickly. In practice, though, you really should never eat less than 800 calories a day without continuous medical supervision. We are actually more comfortable with 1,000 calories. Extremely low-calorie diets are dangerous, because they do not provide the minimum amounts of nutrients and energy you need. They may seriously deplete the body so that normal metabolism is affected. That is why medical supervision is needed if you reduce your calorie intake to less than 800.

* Are all fish low in calories?

The calories in fish depend mainly on its fat content. A serving of fatty fish like mackerel, trout, and salmon has more calories than a similar serving of cod, flounder, or haddock, which are lower in fat. (See the chart "Calories in Fish.")

CALORIES IN FISH*

Finfish	*Calories in 3½ ounces (cooked)*
Bass, striped, broiled	228
Bluefish, filet, baked	160
Cod, broiled	162
Croaker, baked	133
Eel	233

Fishsticks, frozen†	176
Flounder, baked	202
Haddock, broiled	141
Herring, kippered	211
Mackerel, broiled	300
Pompano, broiled	284
Roe, baked	126
Salmon, canned	203
Sardines, canned in oil	311
Trout, cooked	196
Tuna, canned in oil	288
Tuna, canned in water	127

Shellfish

Clams, raw	82
Crab, steamed	93
Lobster, canned	88
Oysters, raw	66
Scallops, steamed	112
Shrimp, canned	80

* Cooked without added fat or coating.
† Commercially prepared with coating.

* Am I fat because my parents were fat?

Overweight seems to be due both to heredity and to environment. Studies show that children with normal-weight parents have only a 14 percent chance of being fat, while if one parent is overweight, the child has as much as a 40 percent chance of being fat. If both parents are overweight the child is even more likely to be fat. Of course, you realize that parents and children have similar eating habits as well as similar genes. Studies show another interesting fact: husbands and wives tend to be similar in their fatness, even shortly after they marry.

While it is true that you may inherit a tendency to be overweight, don't use it as an excuse to explain away your increasing weight.

* Why do women seem to suffer from middle-age spread more than men?

Women are more likely to be overweight than men. Women tend to gain rapidly until ages thirty-five to forty-four but keep on gaining until fifty-five to sixty-four. Men gain too, but their gain levels off sooner—thirty-five to forty-four. No one knows why women continue to gain weight longer than men.

Many overweight women blame it on menopause and the hormone changes at that time. Certainly their bodies' energy needs decrease as they age and women tend to be less active after their children are grown, and this often occurs at the time of menopause. Also women have more fat in their bodies than men, as caloric needs are based on lean body tissue, they need less calories to begin with: women average 25 percent fat, men 15 percent. Both men and women have increasing percentages of fat as they age.

WEIGHT CONTROL EXCHANGES

EXCHANGES FOR CALORIE CONTROL					
	Calories				
Exchange	1,000	1,200	1,500	1,800	2,100
I Milk	2	2	2	2	2
II Vegetables	2	2	2	3	4
III Fruit	3	3	3	3	5
IV Bread	3	5	7	8	10
V Meat	5	6	7	9	10
VI Fat	2	2	4	5	7

* Is there a simple way to plan a reducing diet?

A simple way to plan healthy, reduced-calorie meals is by using food exchange lists. (See the chart "Weight Control Exchanges.") This way you have freedom of choice without tedious calculations. The six lists group foods according to their calories, carbohydrate, fat, and protein content. There are exchange lists for milk, fruit, vegetables, bread, meat, and fat. The bread exchange list really has other foods in it besides bread, such as starchy vegetables, because they are more like bread in their nutrient content. After deciding on the calorie level that is best for you, that calorie level is translated into the number of selections you can pick from each food exchange list every day. You then divide these choices among the meals and snacks you eat. This may sound confusing, but we will explain it carefully.

Suppose you decide, based on what you read in the preceding questions, that you should be eating 1,200 Calories. Look at the chart "Exchanges for Calorie Control." You see that you can have 2 milk exchanges, 2 vegetable exchanges, 3 fruit exchanges, 5 bread exchanges, 6 meat exchanges, and 2 fat exchanges. These exchanges are then divided into meals and snacks. For example:

1,200 CALORIES

EXCHANGE	FOOD
Breakfast	
1 fruit exchange	1 sliced orange
2 bread exchanges	½ cup bran flakes plus 1 slice whole-wheat toast
1 milk exchange	½ cup skim milk*
1 fat exchange	1 teaspoon butter
	Coffee with milk
Lunch	
2 meat exchanges	Open-faced tuna sandwich
1 bread exchange	with lettuce and tomatoes
1 vegetable exchange	and 1 teaspoon
1 fat exchange	mayonnaise
	Coffee or tea or club soda
Dinner	
3 meat exchanges	½ chicken breast
1 vegetable exchange	½ cup green beans
1 bread exchange	½ cup rice
1 fruit exchange	½ cup fruit salad
	Tea or coffee

---

* Remains of 1 cup skim milk can be used in coffee or tea throughout the day.

EXCHANGE	FOOD
Snack I	
1 milk exchange	1 glass skim milk
1 bread exchange	½ large corn muffin
Snack II	
1 fruit exchange	1 apple
1 meat exchange	1 cube cheese

* Is this daily menu of three meals and two snacks one you can live with?

If it isn't, you can borrow from either of the snacks to add to any meal. You can also save some food from a meal to eat later. While this switching around is fine, *don't skip any meals.* That will only set you up for gorging next time you eat.

If you have a sweet tooth and want sugar in your beverages or on your cereal, or jelly on your toast, it's possible. Instead of eating the meat exchange (1 cube of cheese) in Snack II, you can use those calories (about 70) to add some sweetening throughout the day. Four teaspoons of sugar or jelly equals the calories in the meat exchange.

Below are substitutes for Snack I and Snack II to add variety to your menus.

All of the following may be eaten as a substitute for Snack I:

¾ cup skim milk vanilla
   yogurt
½ cup vanilla pudding
½ cup custard
½ cup ice cream
½ cup sherbet
 1 brownie (2 inches square)

1 plain doughnut
½ cup rice pudding with
   raisins
4 ounces Chablis plus 10
   cheese snack crackers
1 apple plus 1 tablespoon
   peanut butter

All of the following may be eaten as a substitute for Snack II:

 6 walnuts plus 1 ounce cheese
½ cup Jell-O plus ¼ cup berries

1 slice raisin bread plus 1 tablespoon cream cheese
6 ounces ginger ale plus ¾ cup popcorn
2 raw carrots plus 7 raw celery stalks
30 fresh cherries
2 chocolate chip cookies
1 pint strawberries
9 ounces Coke
1 large banana

Weight Control Exchanges*

I   Milk Exchanges—1 cup of any of the following equals 1 exchange

> skim or nonfat milk
> plain skim milk yogurt
> buttermilk made from skim milk

If you prefer 2% fat or whole milk you must subtract a fat exchange from that day.

II   Vegetable Exchange—1 cup of any of the following equals 1 exchange

asparagus	mushrooms
bamboo shoots	okra
bean sprouts	onions
beets	pumpkin
broccoli	rhubarb
Brussels sprouts	rutabaga
cabbage	sauerkraut
carrots	string beans, green or yellow
cauliflower	summer squash
celery	tomatoes
cucumber	tomato juice
eggplant	vegetable juice cocktail
green pepper	vegetable soup, undiluted
greens: beet, chard, escarole,	water chestnuts
collard, dandelion, kale, mustard, spinach, turnip	zucchini

* Weight Control Exchanges are based on the 1976 modification of the Exchange System of the American Dietetic Association and American Diabetes Association. They are to be used for weight control only, and not for use by diabetics.

The following raw vegetables can be used as desired:

chicory	lettuce
Chinese cabbage	parsley
endive	radishes
escarole	watercress

III   FRUIT EXCHANGES

(Fruit and amount)	*(No. of exchanges)*
apple	2
⅔ cup apple juice	2
½ cup applesauce	1
2 apricots	1
4 halves dried apricots	1
1 banana	2
½ cup blackberries	1
½ cup blueberries	1
½ cup raspberries	1
¾ cup strawberries	1
10 cherries	1
⅔ cup cider	2
4 dates	2
2 figs	2
½ grapefruit	1
½ cup grapefruit juice	1
12 grapes	1
½ cup grape juice	2
⅔ whole guava	1
3 fresh litchi nuts	1
½ mango	1
¼ cantaloupe	1
⅛ honeydew	1
2-inch wedge Cranshaw	1
2 kumquats	1
1 cup watermelon	1
1 nectarine	1
1 orange	1
½ cup orange juice	1
¾ cup papaya	1

(Fruit and amount)	(No. of exchanges)
1 peach	1
1 pear	1
1 persimmon	1
½ cup pineapple	1
⅔ cup pineapple juice	2
2 plums	1
4 prunes	2
½ cup prune juice	2
2 tablespoons raisins	1
tangerine	1

IV BREAD EXCHANGES (cereal, crackers, starchy vegetables)

(Food and amount)	(No. of exchanges)
1 slice bread, any type	1
1 bagel	2
1 English muffin	2
1 hard roll	2
1 frankfurter or hamburger roll	2
1 tortilla	1
½ to ¾ cup dry unsweetened cereal	1
1 cup unsweetened puffed cereal	1
½ cup rice, barley, cornmeal, oatmeal, cooked cereal	1
½ cup pasta, spaghetti, noodles, macaroni	1
½ cup hominy	1
2 cups popcorn	1
¼ cup wheat germ	1
2 graham crackers	1
1 matzoh	2
4 melba toast	1
½ cup oyster crackers	1
25 pretzel sticks (thin)	1
3 Rye-Krisp	1
6 saltines	1
6 small vanilla wafers	1

(Food and amount)	*(No. of exchanges)*
⅓ cup corn	1
½ cup lentils	1
½ cup beans, any variety	1
⅔ cup parsnips	1
½ cup peas	1
1 small boiled potato	1
½ cup mashed potato	1
½ cup winter (acorn) squash	1
½ cup sweet potato (yams)	2
1 biscuit†	1
1 large corn muffin†	2
4 9-inch breadsticks	1
3-inch cube sponge cake	2
1 pita bread (large size)	2
¼ cup bulgur	2
5 Ritz crackers†	1
1 pancake†	1
1 waffle†	1

† All foods do not fit neatly into the exchange lists. When these bread exchanges are eaten you must add 1 fat exchange. For example: 1 biscuit equals 1 bread exchange plus 1 fat exchange.

V   MEAT EXCHANGES (incl. meat, fish, poultry, eggs, beans)

1 ounce ground round	1
1 ounce pork (loin, butt, chops)	1
1 ounce boiled ham	1
1 ounce Canadian bacon	1
1 ounce liver	1
1 ounce flank steak‡	1
1 ounce leg of lamb‡	1
1 ounce poultry, without skin‡	1
1 ounce brisket§	1
1 ounce corned beef§	1
1 ounce hamburger§	1
1 ounce club steak§	1
1 ounce pork sparerib§	1
1 ounce deviled ham§	1
1 slice luncheon meat§	1
1 small frankfurter§	1
1 ounce fish (fresh or frozen)‡	1

(Food and amount)	*(No. of exchanges)*
¼ cup tuna (water pack)‡	1
¼ cup salmon mackerel‡	1
1 ounce shellfish‡	1
3 sardines	1
⅓ cup low-fat cottage cheese	1
¼ cup creamed cottage cheese	1
¼ cup ricotta cheese	1
1 ounce American cheese, mozzarella, farmer's, edam, camembert, Liederkranz, feta	1
3 tablespoons grated Parmesan	1
½ ounces brick cheese, cheddar, Swiss, muenster, any hard cheese, blue	1
½ cup dried peas and beans	2
1 egg	1
1 tablespoon peanut butter	1
1 cake (2-inch square) tofu	1
¼ cup liquid egg substitute	1

‡ These are lean meat exchanges and the portion size as served can be a little generous.

§ These meat exchanges are higher in fat and the portion size as served should be slightly smaller.

VI FAT EXCHANGES (incl. fat, salad dressing, nuts)

1 teaspoon butter or margarine	1
1 tablespoon French or Italian salad dressing	1
2 teaspoons creamy salad dressing	1
1 tablespoon mayonnaise	1
2 tablespoons sour cream	1
6 walnuts	1
¼ avocado	2
5 olives	1
10 almonds	1
10 peanuts	1
1 strip bacon	1
1 teaspoon vegetable oil	1
1 tablespoon cream cheese	1
1 teaspoon tahini	1
2 teaspoon sesame seeds	1

THE 1,200-CALORIE WEEKLY MENU*

*MONDAY

Breakfast
1 fruit exchange ──────────→ ½ cup grapefruit sections
2 bread exchanges   ½ cup oatmeal
                         1 slice raisin bread
1 fat exchange   1 teaspoon butter
1 milk exchange   1 cup skim milk
                         Coffee

Lunch
2 meat exchanges   2 ounce hamburger on
1 bread exchange   ½ bun
1 vegetable exchange   Sliced tomato
                         Lettuce (free vegetable)
1 fat exchange   1 teaspoon mayonnaise
                         Ice tea, unsweetened

Dinner
3 meat exchanges   3 ounces broiled flounder
1 vegetable exchange   1 cup French-style green beans
1 bread exchange   ½ cup mashed potatoes
1 fruit exchange   1 baked apple
                         Coffee

Snack I
1 milk exchange   1 cup skim milk
1 bread exchange   2 graham crackers

Snack II
1 fruit exchange   1 pear spread with
                         4 tbsp. cottage cheese
1 meat exchange

* Add 2 bread exchanges, 2 fat exchanges, and 1 meat exchange to convert this plan to a 1,500-calorie diet.

*TUESDAY

Breakfast

1 fruit exchange⟶	1 tangerine
2 bread exchanges	1 bagel
1 fat exchange	1 teaspoon butter
1 milk exchange	1 cup skim milk
	Coffee

Lunch

2 meat exchanges	Open-face grilled cheese
1 bread exchange	sandwich
1 vegetable exchange	Green salad with carrot, celery,
	lettuce, and radishes
1 fat exchange	1 tablespoon Italian dressing
	Tea

Dinner

3 meat exchanges	3 ounces roast beef
1 vegetable exchange	1 cup cauliflower
1 bread exchange	1 potato
1 fruit exchange	½ cup crushed pineapple
	Coffee

Snack I

1 milk exchange	1 cup skim milk
1 bread exchange	¾ cup cold cereal

Snack II

1 fruit exchange	⅓ cup apple juice
1 meat exchange	1 tablespoon peanut butter on
	3 saltines†

---

† See snack substitutes in Weight Control Exchanges section, under the Question "Is this daily menu of three meals and two snacks one you can live with?"

*WEDNESDAY

Breakfast
1 fruit exchange ──────────► 1 banana‡
2 bread exchanges   1 cup puffed rice
                                1 slice whole-wheat bread
1 fat exchange   1 teaspoon butter
1 milk exchange   1 cup skim milk
                                Coffee

Lunch
2 meat exchanges   ½ cup creamed cottage cheese
                                    on a bed of greens (free)
1 vegetable exchange   ½ cup raw mixed vegetables
1 bread exchange   1 biscuit
1 fat exchange   Needed for biscuit
                                Club soda with lime

Dinner
3 meat exchanges   3 ounces Canadian bacon
1 vegetable exchange   1 cup cucumber-onion salad
                                    with vinegar
1 bread exchange   ½ cup winter squash
1 fruit exchange   1 fresh peach
                                Coffee

Snack I
1 milk exchange   1 cup yogurt
1 bread exchange   ¼ cup wheat germ

Snack II
1 fruit exchange   Borrowed for breakfast
1 meat exchange   1 cube American cheese

*THURSDAY

Breakfast
1 fruit exchange   ½ cup orange juice
2 bread exchanges   ½ cup Wheatena
                                1 slice toast
1 fat exchange   1 teaspoon butter
1 milk exchange   1 cup skim milk
                                Coffee

‡ Exchange borrowed from a snack.

Lunch

2 meat exchanges ─────────▶ ½ cup salmon salad with
                              mayonnaise on a bed of
                              greens (free)
1 bread exchange   1 slice pumpernickel bread
1 vegetable exchange   1 cup marinated broccoli
1 fat exchange   Needed for salmon salad
                              Coffee

Dinner

3 meat exchanges   1 broiled chicken leg and thigh
1 vegetable exchange   1 cup steamed zucchini
1 bread exchange   ½ cup noodles
1 fruit exchange   1 small bunch of grapes
                              Tea

Snack I

1 milk exchange   ½ cup ice cream†
1 bread exchange   Borrowed for ice cream

Snack II

1 fruit exchange   ⅛ honeydew melon
1 meat exchange   1 ounce ham

*FRIDAY

Breakfast

1 fruit exchange   ¼ cantaloupe
2 bread exchanges   1 English muffin
1 fat exchange   1 tablespoon cream cheese
1 milk exchange   1 cup skim milk
                              Coffee

Lunch

2 meat exchanges   Open-face ham and cheese
1 bread exchange   sandwich
1 vegetable exchange   1 cup coleslaw
1 fat exchange   Needed for coleslaw
                              mineral water

† See snack substitutes in Weight Control Exchanges section, under the Question "Is this daily menu of three meals and two snacks one you can live with?"

Dinner
3 meat exchanges ——————▶ 1 pork chop
1 vegetable exchange   ½ cup sweet potato‡
1 bread exchange   ½ cup peas
1 fuit exchange   ½ cup applesauce
                            Tea

Snack I
1 milk exchange   1 cup skim milk
1 bread exchange   Borrowed for dinner
                            Tea

Snack II
1 fruit exchange   2 chopped dates
1 meat exchange   1 ounce ricotta cheese

*SATURDAY

Breakfast
1 fruit exchange   2 tablespoons raisins
2 bread exchanges   ¾ cup cornflakes
                            1 slice rye bread
1 fat exchange   1 teaspoon butter
1 milk exchange   1 cup skim milk

Lunch
2 meat exchanges   Open-face sliced turkey
1 bread exchange   on rye with Russian dressing
1 vegetable exchange   Green pepper and carrot sticks
1 fat exchange   Need for sandwich
                            Tea

Dinner
3 meat exchanges   3 ounces poached cod
1 bread exchange   ½ cup spaghetti and marinara
                                sauce
1 vegetable exchange   Greens and Zero Dressing (See
                                recipe Chapter 8)
1 fruit exchange   4 apricot halves
                            Coffee

‡ Exchange borrowed from a snack.

Snack I
1 milk exchange————————▶1 cup skim milk
1 bread exchange   6 small vanilla wafers

Snack II
1 fruit exchange   ¾ cup popcorn
1 meat exchange   6 ounces ginger ale†

*SUNDAY

Breakfast
1 fruit exchange   1 fresh pear
2 bread exchanges   2 waffles
1 fat exchange   1 strip crisp bacon
                                 1½ tablespoon syrup*
1 milk exchange   1 cup skim milk

Lunch
2 meat exchanges   English muffin pizza: 2 ounce
                                     mozzarella on 1 whole
                                     muffin‡

2 bread exchange   ½ cup tomato sauce
1 vegetable exchange   1 tablespoon French dressing
1 fat exchange   on greens
                                 Coffee

Dinner
3 meat exchanges   3 ounces flank steak
1 vegetable exchange   1 cup spinach
1 bread exchange   ½ cup winter squash
1 fruit exchange   ¾ cup strawberries
                                 Ice tea

* For those with a sweet tooth, occasionally the calories from 1 meat exchange may be borrowed i.e. syrup for breakfast, see page 345.

† See snack substitutes in Weight Control Exchanges section, under the Question "Is this daily menu of three meals and two snacks one you can live with?"

‡ Exchange borrowed from a snack.

*SUNDAY (cont.)

Snack I

1 milk exchange ─────────→ 1 cup frozen yogurt

1 bread exchange   Borrowed for lunch

Snack II

1 fruit exchange   ½ cup grapefruit juice

1 meat exchange   Borrowed for breakfast

DIETING

✳ How can I stick to my diet when eating out?

It can be done, you simply have to read the menu a little more carefully. Don't rush to order, and don't order a complete dinner. Even though it is more economical, you may be getting more food than you want or need. Order á la carte. Choose foods that are simply prepared, baked and broiled, ask for plain dishes rather than mixtures like casseroles. Request the salad dressing, sour cream, gravy, or sauce on the side so you can have more control.

When you are waiting to be served, or sometimes even before you have ordered, rolls, butter, and other nibbles are brought to the table. Limit your before-meal eating to an *unbuttered* roll, some vegetables without dip, or small amounts of pickled relishes.

Here are some suggestions for ordering:

• *Appetizer.* Choose tomato juice, half grapefruit, melon wedge, or fruit cup. They are refreshing and low in calories. Clams on the half shell and seafood cocktails are also fine, but use the red cocktail sauce, not a creamy dressing. Limit salad dressing to one tablespoon or less. Salad, dressed with vinegar or lemon, makes a fine appetizer.

• *Soup.* Choose a clear soup like chicken, a tomato-based vegetable, or Manhattan clam chowder. Stay away from creamed soups like bisques or New England clam chowder or pureed vegetable.

• _Main dish_. Choose broiled, boiled, roasted, poached, or steamed foods in place of fried or sautéed. To cut calories even further, you can ask that fish, meat, and poultry be prepared without added butter. Have the gravy or sauce served separately "on the side" so that you can add a small amount.

• _Vegetables_. Choose baked potatoes; you can add a small amount of sour cream if you like. Plain boiled or steamed vegetables are usually available. Don't eat those prepared with sauces or creamed, french fried, or batter dipped and deep fried. If there are no suitable vegetables, ask for another salad.

• _Dessert_. This is often a temptation. If you will not be satisfied with a fruit cup, berries, melon, or a baked apple, why not order a "small" dish of sherbert or plain ice cream, or split an order of plain cake with a companion. If you are eating alone, just leave some over. It's not so bad to waste a little food; it's worse to overeat.

• _Beverage_. Tea or coffee are fine. Ask for regular milk in place of cream. Skim milk is a good choice too, and many restaurants offer it. Soft drinks are very high in sugar so that if you want one _occasionally_, drink a small amount.

• _Alcohol_. Choose light beer in place of regular and limit that to one or two glasses. Mixed drinks like diaquiris, Tom Collinses, and martinis, as well as liqueurs (cordials) and brandy are high in calories and should not be ordered. White wine, dry sherry, and dry red wine all have fewer calories.

It may take a little planning, but it's worth it to enjoy an evening out without sabotaging your diet plans.

* How can I tell how much food I should eat for a portion?

It's easy to visualize the portion size for some foods like a glass of milk, or a slice of bread or even an apple or an orange. A half cup of vegetables is the usual portion eaten. Some other foods are a little harder to portion out. Three to four ounces of cooked meat, fish, or poultry is a normal portion, although restaurants often serve much larger amounts. To help you estimate the amount of meat in a portion, see the table "Portion Sizes of Meat."

Most people tend to eat large amounts of rice, noodles, and spaghetti. One half cup is the portion size referred to in diet plans. If you usually eat more than this you may actually be eating two or more portions. (See the section on Weight Control Exchanges for a guide to average portion sizes.)

PORTION SIZES OF MEAT			
Meat	*This thickness*	*Dimensions*	*Calories*
Hamburger, lean	|←¾″→|	3¼″ × 2¼″	185
Roast beef, lean	→|¼″|←	3¾″ × 2″	70
Meatloaf	|←½″→|	2¾″ × 1¾″	85
Pork chop (meat only)	|←½″→|	3¼″ × 1½″	115
Veal cutlet	|←½″→|	4⅛″ × 2¼″	185
Turkey, white meat	→|¼″|←	4″ × 2″	75

✳ What are some good snacks to eat when I am dieting?

Fresh fruits and vegetables are obvious choices. Also fruit canned in its own juice, not in syrup, is good. Small amounts of dried fruit—a small handful of raisins or two or three prunes help satisfy a sweet tooth.

Popcorn, unbuttered of course, is good since it is filling and very low in calories—only 25 in a cupful. Rice cakes are satisfyingly chewy and only 40 calories each. We enjoy a slice of whole-grain raisin bread—no spread needed—with a cup of tea as a delicious pick-me-up. See the chart "Snacks—100 Calories or Less" for many suggestions.

✳ Will a diuretic help me lose weight?

It only seems that way. While it is true you will weigh less after taking a diuretic (also called a "water pill"), it is only a loss of water and minerals. This loss shows that you have dehydrated your body, not lost any fat. Adequate water and mineral content is needed for normal body functions. As soon as you stop taking the water pills the body will again regain its normal water level and the weight you thought lost will be back. Diuretics should be used only for treatment of medical problems.

SNACKS—100 CALORIES OR LESS

Breads

	Calories
Whole-wheat bread, 1 slice with 1 teaspoon jelly	73
Saltines, 2, with 2 teaspoons peanut butter	88
Bagel, ½ toasted with 1 teaspoon jam	100
Graham crackers, 2	100

Fruits

Strawberries, 10 with ½ cup skim milk yogurt	77
Apple, 1	87
Blueberries, 1⅓ cup	87
Cantaloupe, ¾ of a melon	90
Grapefruit, 1 whole	82
Banana, 1 small	90

Miscellaneous

Tossed salad with 1 tablespoon dressing	80
Potato chips, 8	99
Pretzels, small, 3 ring, 9	99
Coffee with milk and 1 teaspoon sugar	35

Sweets

Caramels, 2	76
Marshmallows, 4	100
Fig Newtons, 2	100
Oreos, 2	100
Pound cake, 1 small piece	100
Vanilla ice cream, ⅓ cup plus a few (3 or 4) nuts	100
Gingerbread, 1 small piece	100

Some fad diets include vitamin B_6 along with seaweed and some other things. This is said to act like a diuretic and make you lose weight faster. There is no truth to this. While caffeine and alcohol act as diuretics, no food or vitamin does. We do not recommend the use of diuretics for weight control.

* Are the foods labeled "lite" good to eat when you are trying to lose weight?

Some snack foods, salad dressings, canned fruits, even beer and wine are now produced with about one-third less calories than normal. These foods are called "light" or "lite"—a new term not yet legally defined by federal labeling regulations. That is why you must read the label to see how many calories you are saving by eating these foods.

Under present regulations, foods called "reduced calorie" must contain one-third less calories than the comparable food, while "low-calorie" foods must contain no more than 40 calories a serving. These are standardized definitions. The description "lite" might be used on food even if it has only a few calories less than the regular version.

Check the labels, then try the new lower calorie foods to see if you enjoy them. If you do, they would be a way to reduce calorie intake if you don't increase the amount of the food you eat.

* Can liquid meals help me lose weight?

Any time you eat fewer calories than you need you will lose weight. It doesn't make much difference what form these calories are in—liquid or solid. If you want to lose a few pounds, using a liquid meal to replace a regular meal is all right. Be sure to choose one that is balanced, such as Metrecal or Carnation Slender or Carnation Instant Breakfast. Don't use the liquid protein supplements as they may be dangerous. (See the question "Is the liquid protein diet safe?" in this section.)

Although the prepared liquid meals are calorie convenient and may be appealing at first, they soon become monotonous. Another disadvantage is that they may cause constipation because they lack fiber. In any case, you are not likely to continue using the liquid meals for very long. When you stop, you are bound to regain any weight you lost. You did not change your behavior about food—the way you eat—you changed only what you ate. That method will not lead to permanent weight loss.

* I have a friend who told me she vomits after a big meal or a party to help control her weight. What do you think of this?

If your friend does this regularly she may be suffering from bulimia. This condition—binge eating, followed by self-induced vomiting—is an eating disorder. Although the practice is ancient (wealthy Romans feasted, visited a vomitorium to purge, and returned to feast some more) bulimia has only recently been categorized as a medical condition. Today the practice may be more widespread than we realize. Celebrities admit to using this as a means of weight control. Many vomit so that they may enjoy eating without worrying about the calories.

It may seem tempting, but don't do it! Bulimiacs need medical, psychological, and dietary treatment. Repeated self-induced vomiting is dangerous, causing sore throat, dental decay, esophageal irritation, dehydration, fatigue, and even stomach rupture.

If you want to control your weight, you need to learn to control your food intake. Eating an occasional big meal or overeating at a party will not cause a weight gain as long as you regularly eat sensibly and exercise.

* Will eating too much salt make me gain weight?

No, not really. Because even though you may weigh more after eating salty food, it is only temporary. As soon as you drink enough water to carry the salt out of the body, the extra weight will be gone. Some people take a little longer to get rid of the salt and water. Hormonal changes in women during the menstrual cycle may interfere and slow down the process. But, in spite of this, eating salt does not cause a permanent weight gain.

EXERCISE

* Do I have to exercise to lose weight?

It's not absolutely essential, but it really helps. You may be discouraged when you hear that if you weigh 155 pounds, you would have to walk more than an hour to use up the calories in a single hamburger. While that is true, it is only part of the story. The calories you use up in exercise accumulate so that just a little extra exercise a few times during the day adds up. You don't have to take that hour walk all at one time. Exercise provides a bonus. It increases the amount of energy that is used even after you finish exercising. Your metabolic rate and the calories you burn are higher for hours after—sort of like your motor idling at a higher level.

Exercise has other advantages. It improves your muscles, heart, and lungs. Also, weight lost from exercise is mainly fat, not water or muscle, and fat is what you want to lose. And if this isn't enough, exercise can be enjoyable, more fun for most people than dieting is.

Regular exercise is just as important to your health as good food. Walking is popular and appropriate for all ages. You may be surprised to hear walking a mile burns up nearly as many calories as if you jogged it!

One note of caution: If you are over thirty-five and are starting to exercise, a physical exam is recommended.

* If I want to lose weight do I have to exercise every day?

If you want to be successful in losing weight and keeping it off, it is very helpful to exercise. When you lose weight by calorie restriction alone, 25 percent of the loss is muscle. When and if you regain this weight it will be entirely fat. That way you can wind up with more fat than you had when you started. This increased fat can make you more inactive so that you might gain even more. When you exercise in addition to cutting calories you will lose fat and at the same time increase your muscle size.

Regular exercise helps, but it doesn't have to be daily. You should aim for about three one-hour sessions each week. This will have additional benefits of toning muscles, increasing your heart's efficiency, raising your HDL level, and enhancing your feeling of well-being as it improves your shape. And last but not least, it takes up time that might have been spent eating.

* Doesn't exercise increase your appetite?

No, it actually may reduce it. It seems that a certain amount of activity is needed to regulate appetite. Studies show that for most of us, moderate exercise done for extended periods will cause no change in the amounts of food we eat. On the other hand, vigorous exercise for shorter periods has been shown to suppress appetite. Another bonus is that exercise reduces tension and depression that might prompt you to eat when you are not hungry.

* How can I judge my level of daily activity?

We are often asked this question. It may be hard to tell if you are sedentary, moderately active, or very active. Just because you seem to be on the go all day doesn't mean you are really "active." The "Weight and Activity Profile" on page 186 will help you judge your own daily activity level.

* Is it really healthier to be a little underweight?

Insurance company studies show that people who weigh 5 to 15 percent less than average live longer and have fewer debilitating illnesses. (Of course that is true only if the person has no other health problem.) Other researchers report that it is healthier to be slightly over average (note the word *slightly*).

While researchers debate, what is certain is that if you are overweight, you are more likely to have high blood pressure, diabetes, heart disease, and other illnesses. If you already suffer from these disorders, treatment often includes weight loss.

RATE YOURSELF:

	Weight and Activity Profile			
	+2	**+1**	**0**	**Points**
1. In the last year, your weight has:	been stable	increased 5 pounds or less	increased more than 5 pounds	_____
2. If your weight at age 25 was ideal, you are now:	the same weight	10 percent heavier	20 percent heavier	_____
3. Each day you walk a total of:	5 miles or more	3 miles or more	less than 1 mile	_____
4. Each day you climb a total of:	10 or more staircases	5 or more staircases	less than 1 staircase	_____
5. Each week you exercise:	½ hour every other day	½ hour less than 3 times a week	not at all	_____

Total points _____

8–10 = You are in excellent shape
5–7 = You are in fair shape
Under 5 = You are in poor shape

Rather than waiting for the researchers to agree on what is the optimum weight, we feel that you can decide on the best weight for yourself—the weight where you feel and look best. It will probably fall within 5 to 10 percent of desirable weight.

The *set point* theory of body weight states that each person has a certain weight that his body is set to maintain. This would explain how quickly dieters can return to their previous weight after going off a diet. This may also explain how otherwise healthy people may maintain their weight at a level below normal. If you are a little underweight without dieting, then your body's set point may simply be lower than that of other people's.

* Will joining a weight-reducing group help?

Some people enjoy the camaraderie and mutual support they get from attending weekly sessions with others who, like themselves, are trying to lose weight. Some find it helpful to have a monitor who can encourage their success and scold their failure. If you feel that you can benefit from this group approach to weight loss, why not try it?

Before choosing a group, be sure to read the literature that describes the program. That will help you to pick a group you will be comfortable with. You also should check the kind of diet they use so that you can be sure it is a sound one you can live with. Some of the programs use diets that are extremely low in calories (under 1,000 daily) and also very low in carbohydrates. You would be safer and more likely to have long-term success with a program that uses a balanced diet that is moderately restricted in calories.

Many programs now combine behavior modification techniques with a diet plan and this is a good approach. Some programs, though, emphasize the psychological aspects of overweight but suggest poor eating plans. Choose one that offers sound all-around help, such as Weight Watchers.

UNSAFE DIETING

* What is phenylpropanolamine? I see it listed as an ingredient in diet pills.

Phenylpropanolamine (PPA) is an ingredient in over-the-counter diet pills like Dietac, Prolamine, Dexatrim, Appedrine, Ayds, and Control. This stimulant, which is also a drug used as a nasal decongestant, seems to work by reducing your appetite while at the same time dulling your senses of taste and smell. Food doesn't taste as good as it usually does after you take PPA.

While the products seem to be slightly helpful for some in

losing weight, they may be dangerous for people with high blood pressure or heart disease. Some of the preparations are labeled with warnings for those with high blood pressure, heart disease, diabetes, or thyroid disease. Others warn against use by pregnant women or nursing mothers and children under eighteen.

There is evidence that when users stop taking the appetite suppressants there is a rebound and weight is regained faster than after other types of diets. While the pills, in the amounts recommended, may not be dangerous for normal, healthy adults, they act only as a crutch and are not effective in the long run. They are not a replacement for sound diet and regular exercise.

* Is fasting a safe way to lose weight?

It isn't when you do it yourself. A one-day fast is safe for healthy people, but fasting for longer than that may not be. Fasting causes body changes—there is a loss of water and minerals. Lean body tissue (muscles) are used along with fat stores to provide energy. The body begins to waste. Body fat lost during fasting is no more than what you would lose on a low-calorie diet. Substances are formed that cannot be metabolized to energy because there is no carbohydrate available. This upsets the acid-base balance in the body and also can cause gout in people who are susceptible. Bad breath, headache, light-headedness, and nausea are other effects.

Fasting is dangerous; it is definitely not a do-it-yourself approach to losing weight. (For more information about fasting see the question "Is fasting a good way to rid my body of poisons?" in Chapter 10.)

* Will a laxative help me lose weight?

Some people take laxatives after every meal in the hope that it will keep them from absorbing the food they have just eaten. While it can do this to some extent, it will also cause a loss of water and minerals in the diarrhea that results. This is not a safe way to reduce.

* Is the liquid protein diet safe?

No, it is not. There have been a number of deaths from abnormal heart rhythms in people who were taking liquid protein (amino acid) preparations and no other food. No one is sure exactly what caused the deaths, but in most cases the dieters had no history of heart disease and some were under a doctor's supervision as well.

It may be tempting to diet with measured amounts of protein mixtures and not have to deal with choosing regular foods. But besides being dangerous, it is not realistic. It's not likely that you would want to live on liquid protein with little or no other food for more than a month or so. Headaches, sluggishness, gas, and bad breath are common complaints. Liquid protein and other protein products sold for use in weight reduction are now required to be labeled with warnings.

* Will those special belts they sell to reduce your waistline work?

They only seem to work by causing water loss or muscle contractions. No fat is lost. Unfortunately, this water loss is temporary. Rubber or plastic body wraps for legs, chins, and necks and sauna suits work on the same principle—they cause shrinkage and weight loss by removing water from the skin. For most, these devices are merely a waste of money, but for people with diabetes, varicose veins, or other circulation problems, the wraps could be dangerous.

* My friend says she has finally lost weight on the Beverly Hills Diet, is this really good?

Like other fad diets that enjoy brief periods of popularity, you can lose weight on the Beverly Hills Diet. But although it is novel (and maybe fun at first), it will not help you to lose weight and keep it off.

For the first ten days of the diet, nothing but fruit is eaten. Besides getting tired of so much fruit, you may also develop diarrhea. This diarrhea is uncomfortable and unpleasant and depletes your body of nutrients. Fruit is high in sugar and low in protein and fats. After the initial ten days, you begin to add bread and vegetables. Meat or fish is not eaten until the nineteenth day. Obviously the diet does not provide the nutrients you need for good health. For some, who do not metabolize sugar normally, the diet may be risky.

Excess eating is encouraged as huge portions of food are suggested—one-half pound of prunes, five pounds of grapes. Even if you could possibly eat that much, would you want to?

Besides the bizarre nature of the diet, the author offers lots of misinformation about digestion. For example, she says that when your body does not process food, the food turns into fat. Actually, food that is not digested is never really inside the body. It remains in the digestive tract, which keeps undigested food from entering the body's cells and tissues. So the body cannot turn this food into fat—or anything else for that matter. Undigested food is passed out of the body in your stool.

Your friend has seen the initial loss—mainly water—from the diet. She is doomed to failure because following a novel diet like this one is fun for a while but quickly becomes tiresome. The dieter resumes eating usual foods before long. That results in the lost weight coming back quickly, often with a little extra.

* Is the Scarsdale Diet a good one?

The Scarsdale Diet is just another name for the low-carbohydrate, high-protein, high-fat diet that appears from time to time under a variety of names. Atkins, Air Force, Stillman Quick-Weight Loss, Mayo, and Calories Don't Count are similar diets that were popular in the past and surely there will be more in the future.

In the Scarsdale Diet you are given a week of menus to follow, but the amounts of food to be eaten are not given. Obviously that's not a good approach. It is almost license to stuff yourself.

The low-carbohydrate content of the diet leads to loss of water, which results in a rapid weight loss. As the water is lost it carries with it vitamins and minerals that are not easily replaced by the limited foods permitted. Because it is water lost and not fat, the weight loss is regained as soon as regular eating is resumed.

Besides not being effective, a low-carbohydrate diet is not a good choice for other reasons. Lack of carbohydrate leads to the accumulation of ketones (ketones are formed when fat is incompletely metabolized due to a lack of carbohydrate) in the body, which can make you feel nauseous, tired, and even dizzy. The larger amount of fat and protein in this diet is not healthy either. It can lead to cardiovascular disease, certain types of cancer, and bone loss.

Last, but really not the least, a diet that restricts carbohydrate foods reduces the amount of fiber. You have less to chew on, to fill your stomach with and to soften your bowels. Besides, carbohydrate foods, such as bread, pasta, and potatoes taste good, are low in calories (when not served spread with fat), and have been shown to promote weight loss. An eight-week study in which subjects ate twelve slices of high fiber bread a day resulted in an average weight loss of almost twenty pounds.

Low-carbohydrate diets like the Scarsdale Diet can give you a short-term loss of weight but are useless for a sustained weight loss.

* What is the Cambridge Diet?

This is an extremely low-calorie diet, that uses a flavored powder mixed with water drunk three times a day. The powder used is sold through the Cambridge Plan. It provides only 330 calories per day from 31 grams protein, 44 grams carbohydrate, and 3 grams of fat. Claims are made that it provides the Recommended Dietary Allowances for all essential vitamins and minerals. However, several followers of the diet have been hospitalized for heart irregularities believed due to mineral imbalances. Any diet containing so few calories is dangerous. There should be continuous medical supervision when following it. In fact, such a warning appears on the Cambridge Plan product labels, but that, in itself, is no assurance that users will seek medical supervision.

* What kind of operation is done to help you lose weight?

About twenty thousand extremely obese Americans have had an intestinal bypass operation in an attempt to lose weight. Unfortunately, after surgery, which ties off the major portion of the intestine, about 15 percent develop arthritis, kidney or liver damage, and a small percentage die. Researchers now recommend that this procedure be used rarely, if at all.

Newer methods used to treat gross obesity are stapling off a portion of the stomach or wrapping the stomach with plastic mesh to lessen its capacity. Another method is to place a balloon in the abdomen above the stomach, which compresses the stomach so the person will eat less. Because these treatments are so new, there is no way to judge their long-term benefits.

* What are starch blockers?

Starch blockers are diet aids sold under a variety of names—Sta-Trim, A.A.I., Amylex, Colorex, S.L.P.C., Starch-Block—made from a protein derivative of raw beans. Promoters claim these products will allow you to eat and enjoy carbohydrate foods without digesting and absorbing starch calories. Sounds good but the picture is not all rosy. Large amounts of undigested starch cause gas, bloating, cramps and diarrhea. These side effects alone could cut down on eating and calorie intake. If you are encouraged to eat more starch because you are taking a starch blocker, you probably will be eating less fat and fatty protein and consequently be taking in less calories that can result in weight loss.

There have been reports of medical crises caused by the use of these pills. Officials of the Food and Drug Administration believe there is inadequate support of weight loss claims and they are concerned about the safety of long-term use. The future of starch blockers is uncertain. We'd urge caution if you choose to use starch blockers since they don't change eating habits and may be unsafe.

* Can acupuncture help me lose weight?

There have been claims that acupuncture can help people lose weight. The theory is that by inserting needles into the vagus nerve in the outer ear you can stop hunger contractions in the stomach. The person who has been treated will then eat less and lose weight.

If you decide to try this experimental medical procedure, be sure you follow the recommendation of the American Medical Association, which is that acupuncture be performed only by a licensed physician or dentist or under the direct supervision of one.

* What is cellulite?

Cellulite is the name used for the lumpy fat deposits that dimple hips and thighs. It is claimed that this fat is different from regular fat in that it has to be broken up by massage or other methods before you can lose it, even when you diet.

In fact there is no special fat. Fat is fat and it is one and the same. Singling some of it out with a special name for special notice is simply a way for people to make money by offering unique treatments for it.

SUGAR SUBSTITUTES

* When I'm trying to lose weight is fructose better for me than plain sugar?

Fructose, a sugar made from corn (or found naturally in fruits), is sweeter than regular table sugar—sucrose. Because of its sweetness you can use less. In this way you would be getting about 10 percent fewer calories from foods you sweeten with fructose in place of sugar.

Some people believe that fructose is better for those on a diet because it is metabolized slowly and does not require insulin initially the way sugar does. Eating sugar stimulates insulin production, which in turn lowers your blood sugar and makes you feel hungry. Fructose would not have the same effect.

Remember, though, that both sugars contain the same number of calories and will add to your calorie total. So, though fructose may have some slight advantage over regular sugar, you are better off limiting them both.

* Should I use sugar substitutes when I am dieting?

Using calorie-free or low-calorie sugar substitutes like saccharin and aspartame can satisfy your sweet tooth with fewer calories than regular sugar. But some studies have shown that animals eating sugar substitutes ate more food than the animals who ate sugar. This has made some people wonder whether sugar substitutes really are an aid to dieting.

We feel that while these substitutes may help you to eat lower calorie food, they should be used sparingly. Remember that dieting can be successful only when you learn to eat (and enjoy eating) in a more moderate way. Drinking lots of low-calorie soft drinks or eating artificially sweetened desserts will not help you to do this.

* Does saccharin cause cancer?

We have been using saccharin for over eighty years as a sugar substitute in food, drinks, drugs, toothpaste, and mouthwash. It's estimated that we eat 5 to 7 million pounds a year, in diet sodas and the rest in coffee, tea, and as a sweetener in foods. Saccharin seems to pose little trouble to humans since it is not metabolized in the body and passes out through the kidneys almost unchanged. In the mid-seventies, however, saccharin was linked to bladder cancer in rats. By 1977 saccharin was to be banned by the FDA as a carcinogen. The ban was never implemented because the carcinogenic risk was not conclusively established. Instead, a moratorium was set through June 1983 while further research is completed.

In the meantime, saccharin may be used and sold. Are we at risk? Recent research seems to indicate that at the worst, saccharin is a weak carcinogen that does not increase the risk of bladder cancer. Research has not yet determined the risk to other organs or assessed the ill effects of saccharin in heavy users. Heavy use has been defined by Dr. Hoover of the National Cancer Institute as drinking more than four diet sodas a day. Heavy use plus cigarette smoking may increase the carcinogenic effect of saccharin. Until all the results are in, our advice would be to go easy and try to enjoy foods that are less sweet. The chart "Saccharin in Sodas and Sweeteners" will help you determine how much saccharin you use each day.

SACCHARIN IN SODA AND SWEETENERS

Soda	Amount	Milligrams of saccharin
A & W Diet Root Beer	12 ounces	126
Diet Pepsi	12 ounces	125
Diet Rite	12 ounces	144
Diet 7-Up	12 ounces	88
Sugar-Free Sprite	12 ounces	86
Tab	12 ounces	110
Sweetener		
Sucaryl Liquid	⅛ teaspoon	7.6
Sweet 'n Low	1 level teaspoon	20
Sugar Twin	1 level teaspoon	14

* Is there a substitute for saccharin?

After much research and years of testing, a new sweetener, aspartame, derived from protein, has been approved. Sold under the brand name Equal in granular form, it resembles saccharin. Aspartame is very sweet, one packet equals two teaspoons of sugar, and it has no bitter aftertaste. It blends well with food flavors, mellowing the taste of coffee and enhancing the zest of fruit. Aspartame will be used as a sugar substitute or in processed foods like cold breakfast cereals (Quaker Oats Halfsies), chewing gums, instant coffee and tea, gelatin, pudding and pie filling mixes, and nondairy whipped toppings. For now, it will not be used in soda since its flavor fades when stored as a liquid, nor in baking mixes since aspartame is unstable at high temperature.

A low-calorie bulking agent, polydextrose, has also been released for use. It is the first new food additive approved by the FDA in over five years. It is not a sweetener, but it is a low-calorie product that will replace high-calorie sugar or fat in frozen desserts, cakes, and candy. Using polydextrose may reduce calories in some foods up to 50 percent and will allow many new "diet" foods to be developed.

* Is ice milk less fattening than regular ice cream?

Some brands of ice milk labeled 99 PERCENT FAT-FREE may have less calories than regular ice cream. A cup of this ice milk has about 150 calories compared to 250 in ice cream. But you cannot generalize about all kinds of ice milk because some have so much sugar and thickeners added that they have nearly the same calorie content as ordinary ice cream.

Sugar-free ice cream sweetened with sorbitol is calorically equal to regular ice cream. If it is sweetened with fructose, less is used and it may have slightly fewer calories. If sweetened with saccharin, it will be lower too. Look on the labels for calorie information.

Frozen yogurts are often considered low-calorie substitutes for ice cream. Plain vanilla has about 180 calories a cup while the fruit-flavored types average 220 calories. That's not much different from ice cream. Choose types made with skim milk yogurt.

* I have an unusual problem: I'm skinny. How can I gain weight?

You have a problem that makes you the envy of many who wish for a slim figure. If you are in good health, your low weight is simply because you do not eat enough food to permit weight gain. How to eat more food is not simple. Food probably is not of great interest to you.

Time takes care of this problem for many who are too thin in their teens and twenties. They begin to add pounds at middle age. If you don't want to wait for this to happen, or if you are middle-aged and you have not gained, here are some suggestions that may help.

HOW TO GAIN WEIGHT

• Be sure to eat regular meals daily; never skip breakfast or other meals.

• Stop smoking. This will help you gain weight and improve your health as a bonus.

• Exercise daily. This will relax you so that you sleep better and maybe not waste as many calories fidgeting.

• Emphasize high-calorie foods at meals and for between-meal snacks.

• Don't drink liquids with meals, as these will quickly fill you, leaving little room for food.

• Eat snacks between meals and at bedtime. Don't eat so much that you won't be hungry for the next meal or that you won't sleep comfortably.

• Don't eat a lot of bulky foods like salads until you have eaten the main course of your meal.

• Try to eat just a little more than you feel like eating.

• If you are tense at mealtime, rest before eating or try a little wine for an appetizer. This may stimulate your appetite.

8

Diet, High Blood Pressure, and Your Heart

Diseases of the heart and arteries should concern us all. If experience is any guide, more than half of us will die from heart disease. What is worse, one-fourth of everyone who dies from cardiovascular disease is younger than sixty-five. What a waste!

Many researchers are investigating the causes and treatment of cardiovascular diseases. Several factors have been identified that increase the risk. A number of these involve nutrition. In fact, of the three most significant risk factors—elevated cholesterol level, high blood pressure, and cigarette smoking—two can be treated, at least in part, by diet changes. Another risk factor—obesity—also responds to diet.

Authorities have recommended changes in our carbohydrate, fat, fiber, and salt consumption, as well as in the total calories we eat. Often these recommendations are challenged as being based on insufficient evidence, too drastic, and really not appropriate for all Americans. There is much controversy about what constitutes optimum preventive nutrition. While we appreciate the controversial nature of some of these recommendations, we don't think it is wise to wait until all the answers are in before making some moderate changes in what foods and how much we eat.

We feel that most of us would be better off with fewer calories, less fat—both saturated and polyunsaturated—less

198

salt, less sugar, and more fiber. One direct way toward all these ends is to eat more unprocessed and slightly processed foods: use whole-grain cereals and bread often. Use more fresh fruits and vegetables (frozen is a good back-up). Enjoy lean meat, fish, and poultry. Try meat substitutes like skim milk cheeses, soybean curd, dried peas, beans, and lentils. These simple changes can help you to lose weight and save money. Read this chapter to find out how to reduce your risks.

CHOLESTEROL

* Why is a low-fat diet good for me?

Most of us eat much more fat than we need. Fat is a concentrated source of calories that we eat along with other foods, maybe without even noticing. The butter you spread on your toast has almost as many calories as the toast itself. The salad dressing often has many more calories than the salad greens. Reducing excess calories is one reason why a diet low in fat is good, but there are other reasons too.

Recently, diet fat has been linked to cancer of the colon and breast cancer. People who eat more fat are more likely to get these types of cancer. Fat also is a risk factor in the development of atherosclerosis, a major cause of cardiovascular disease, which leads to death from heart attack or stroke.

So you see, there are many advantages to be gained from eating less fat. Working to break the fat-eating habit is worth it.

* Don't I need some fat for good health?

Yes, you do need some fat, but just a little. Most of us eat much more than we need. Americans eat over 40 percent of all their calories as fat. We could be healthy and well fed with much less. In fact, only 5 grams of fat a day would meet our need for essential fatty acids. That's about one teaspoonful. While we aren't suggesting that you limit your fat intake to this amount (it would be almost impossible), we do believe that we all should take steps to limit the amount of fat we eat. Read the other questions in this section for suggestions on how to reduce fat. (Also see "I want to eat less fat. How can I do it?" in Fat section in Chapter 1.)

✻ What are essential fatty acids and why do I need them?

Essential fatty acids, sometimes inaccurately called "vitamin EFA," or "vitamin F," are needed in the diet. Actually, only one of the original three essential fatty acids truly deserves the name: linoleic acid. The other two can be made from it.

Linoleic acid is used to make prostaglandins, hormone-like substances that are important regulators. Linoleic acid is part of the cell membranes around every cell in your body and functions in the metabolism of cholesterol.

A deficiency of essential fatty acid is not something we need to worry about as we have a supply of linoleic acid in the fat stored in our body, and our diet, particularly vegetable oils, supplies plenty. In American diets, 4 to 5 percent of the calories are essential fatty acids and our requirement is only about 1 to 2 percent. It is not necessary to take a fatty acid supplement.

✻ The doctor put my husband on a low-fat diet. What should he eat?

In order to plan low-fat meals and snacks, start thinking about all foods in terms of fat content—both visible and invisible. The fat you can't see in cheddar cheese, for example, is just as important as the more visible fat in butter or margarine.

Here are some low-fat diet suggestions:

LOW-FAT DIET IDEAS

Milk. Use skim milk. Milk labeled SKIM has less than 1 percent fat (that equals 1 gram of fat per cup) and is lower in fat than milk labeled LOW FAT or 1% MILK (also referred to as

"99% fat-free"). Dry Skim Milk is practically fat-free. Two percent milk is becoming more available, and while this is lower in fat than whole milk (3.5 percent fat), it contains more than skim milk. Check the label of yogurt too. Be sure it is made from skim milk.

Avoid coffee whiteners, liquid or powder, used in place of milk or cream. They are high in fat—about equal to the amount in half and half (18%).

Cheese. Use skim milk cheese. Cottage cheese with 1 percent fat is usually available. Other low-fat cheese may be harder to find. Cheese made from partly skimmed milk is still high in fat. See the chart "Fat and Cholesterol in Cheese" to pick low-fat varieties, and the next question. Avoid all hard and soft whole-milk cheeses.

Meat, fish, and poultry. Use poultry and fish often, lean beef, lamb, pork, and veal less often. Cook without added fat—broil, bake, roast, or stew. Pour off and discard meat drippings. (If you wish to use them for gravy, refrigerate first so fat will congeal on top and can be removed easily). Avoid fatty meats like corned beef, sausage, bacon, duck, goose, ham, and fish canned in oil.

Bread. Use all types—enriched white, whole wheat, rye, bran, bagels, English muffins. Avoid sweet rolls, Danish pastry, French toast.

Cereals. Use all kinds—cooked and dry breakfast cereals, also spaghetti, macaroni, rice, and noodles. Avoid granola-type cereals and wheat germ. They are high in fat.

Fruit and vegetables. Use all types, raw or cooked, without added butter or cream. Dried peas and beans are good. Avoid avocados, olives, coconut.

Eggs. Whole eggs should be limited to three a week, cooked without added butter. Egg whites can be used as desired. Two egg whites are equal to one egg in recipes calling for eggs.

Butter, margarine and oil. Butter and margarine are 80 percent fat—and oil is all fat. Use these in very small amounts, two to three tablespoons a day.

Other foods. Sour cream, whipped cream, whipped topping, olives, avocados, coconut, nuts, seeds, chocolate, peanuts, and peanut butter are all high in fat and should be used sparingly.

HINTS. Clear soup is usually lower in fat than cream soup. Use very little of your usual salad dressing. Vinegar or lemon can be used, as can Zero Dressing (see recipe in Special Salad Dressing section in this chapter).

Low fat desserts are gelatin, raw or cooked fruit, fruit whip, sherbet, ices, ice milk, and angel cake. Yogurt is often a good substitute for sour cream, but be careful when cooking with it as it becomes liquid easily. Don't stir it or heat it too much. Use spray shortenings (Pam) to oil any baking pans.

* Is part skim milk cheese better if you are on a low-fat diet?

There is not much difference in the fat content of hard cheese labeled PART SKIM MILK, such as Jarlsberg and regular hard cheese, such as Swiss. That is because although partly skimmed milk has been used initially to make the cheese, additional fat is added in the making. The fat content of a cheese depends most on how much moisture is removed in processing. There are a few types of hard cheese becoming available that are lower in fat. One Danish cheese, Danbo 20 is a good choice. St. Otho, Swiss Lorraine, Lorraine cheddar, and sapsago are others you might try. Sapsago, a green cheese, is only used grated, mixed into other foods. Ask in your local cheese store for other suggestions.

Fresh cheese, like ricotta, cottage, farmer's, pot, and feta cheese are lower in fat. Among these, some are lower than others. While cottage cheese must contain at least 4 percent fat, the low-fat types have only between ½ and 2 percent. They don't taste as creamy but they can be improved with a little low-fat yogurt mixed in.

Ricotta cheese comes in whole milk and skim milk types with the skim variety containing about 8 percent fat and the whole milk 13 percent. Pasta dishes using the skim milk variety are delicious.

Pot cheese and farmer cheese vary in their fat content, as they have not been standardized for labeling.

If you like hard cheese, remember a little can go a long way. When the cheese is used along with pasta, rice, or eaten in small amounts with bread, its high fat content may not be so important. (See the chart below.)

FAT AND CHOLESTEROL IN CHEESE

Cheese	Percent of fat	Milligrams of cholesterol (per ounce)
Cottage, Low-fat 1 percent	1	1
Farmer cheese (Friendship)	1	10
Cottage, creamed	4.5	4
Ricotta, part skim milk	8	7
Ricotta, whole milk	13	14
Mozzarella, part skim milk	16	16
Feta	21	24
Mozzarella, whole milk	22	22
Neufchâtel	23	21
Camembert	24	20
Provolone	27	19
Swiss	27	26
Brie	28	28
Gouda	28	32
Edam	28	25
Blue	28	20
Brick	30	26
Muenster	30	26
Roquefort	31	25
American	31	26
Colby	32	27
Cheddar	33	30
Cream cheese	35	30

* I'm on a low-fat diet and I don't like margarine, what can I do?

Better-Butter is just what you've been looking for. A combination of a polyunsaturated vegetable oil plus the natural, delicious flavor of butter. Better-Butter has the same reduced amount of saturated fat as margarine, but since it spreads so easily and has a butter flavor you tend to use much less than if you were spreading stick margarine or regular butter.

Following is the recipe for one pound of Better-Butter.*

Better Butter

1 cup butter (2 sticks or ½ pound)
½ teaspoon salt (optional)
2 tablespoons water
2 tablespoons dried skim milk
¼ teaspoon powdered lecithin
1 cup safflower, soy, corn or sunflower oil

1. Let butter soften slightly (leave at room temperature about ½ hour). Cut in cubes and whip in blender.
2. Dissolve salt in water, add to butter along with dried skim milk and lecithin; as you blend ingredients slowly pour in oil until mixture is thoroughly combined.
3. Store in refrigerator in a covered container. Makes 1 pound.

1 tablespoon = 111 Calories
17 mg cholesterol

The addition of water, skim milk, and lecithin produces a "butter" that does not separate and stays solid longer at room temperature. Powdered lecithin may be purchased at the health food store. Starting with regular salted butter and adding the oil results in a "butter" with half the sodium content of regular. Since we are always looking for ways to reduce sodium, we prefer not to add the extra ½ teaspoon of salt.

✳ Should I use whipped toppings and coffee creamers?

Even though these products (Cool Whip, Pream, and Cof-fee-mate) may be labeled NONDAIRY, they are high in satu-rated fat. Often coconut or palm (high in saturates) is used or other vegetable fat, which are hardened by *hydrogenization*.

---

* From *Laurel's Kitchen: A Handbook for Vegetarian Cookery and Nutrition* by Laurel Robertson, Carol Flinders, and Bronwen Godfrey, copyright © 1976, by Nilgiri Press, Petaluma, California 94953.

This process saturates the fat and keeps the product fresh. It is better to use skim milk in coffee or try it black.

The whipped cream topping in cans (Reddi-whip) that is made from cream and nonfat milk is 24 percent fat compared to 37 percent fat in heavy whipping cream. So when you whip your own it is higher in fat.

* Can I stick to my low-fat diet if I eat in fast food restaurants?

It isn't easy. A recent analysis of food from three major fast food chains—Burger Chef, Burger King, and McDonald's—showed that most selections were high in fat. In fact, only the shakes and buttered English muffins could be considered moderate in fat, and even in these fat averaged 20 to 30 percent of the calories.

If the fast food restaurant has a salad bar (see following question) and you limit the dressing you use and order broiled meat or fish with a baked potato (sorry, no french fries) or corn on the cob, there is no reason to avoid fast food restaurants. (See the chart "Nutritional Analysis of Fast Foods" in Appendix A for more information.)

* When I eat out and I limit my meal to the salad bar, can I stay on a low-fat diet?

More and more restaurants, both fast food and other, are offering salad bars either as a course in a larger meal or alone with soup and bread. It is possible to eat a low-fat meal by choosing carefully from the salad bar selections.

Stay away from marinated mixtures, slaws with dressing, bacon bits, greasy croutons, sesame seeds, and prepared salad dressings. Pick salad greens, chopped vegetables such as carrots, green pepper, chick-peas, kidney beans, mushrooms, and bean sprouts. Sprinkle your salad with vinegar or a squeeze of lemon and fresh ground pepper. Add unbuttered whole-grain bread and a bowl of soup and you have a delicious, satisfying low-fat meal you can enjoy.

Cholesterol

* What is cholesterol?

Cholesterol is a fat that is part of every cell in your body. Hormones, vitamin D, bile (used for digestion), and sebum (fat that keeps your skin smooth) are all made from cholesterol. So you see, cholesterol is important. You make about two-thirds of the cholesterol you use and get the other third in your food.

The major food source of cholesterol is egg yolk. An average yolk contains about 250 milligrams. Liver, shrimp, heart, kidney, and brains are other rich sources. All meats, milk, fish, and chicken contain cholesterol. There is no cholesterol in vegetables, vegetable oils, fruits, cereals, or grains. (See the chart "Cholesterol in Foods" in this section for the cholesterol content of some common foods.)

* Are triglycerides in the blood the same as cholesterol?

Both triglycerides and cholesterol are fats found in the blood. While both of these fats have been studied as risk factors in heart disease, it seems that cholesterol is more important. That is the reason why it's a good idea for us to eat less cholesterol and saturated fat. Both can lead to higher cholesterol levels in the blood.

Some people have a lot of triglycerides in their blood (150 milligrams percent is considered the upper limit of normal). High triglycerides are treated by reducing weight, eating only a moderate amount of carbohydrate, and reducing the intake or eliminating alcoholic beverages.

* Will a low-cholesterol diet really help me avoid a heart attack?

Yes, more and more we see evidence that eating a diet low in cholesterol and other fats will reduce your chance of having a heart attack.

Because some people have heard that there is no definite proof of the value of eating less cholesterol and fat, they feel that they can continue to eat fatty and cholesterol-rich foods.

They are waiting for some assurance that depriving themselves of their favorite foods would be worth it. The answer appears to be yes! Newer evidence shows that these diet changes are worthwhile.

High blood cholesterol levels are only one of the risk factors for heart attack; there are others you should know about. (See the question "What are the other risk factors for heart attack beside cholesterol?" in this section.)

* I believe my serum cholesterol is high. What foods should I avoid?

Generally, when a person has a serum cholesterol level over 250 milligrams percent, diet is recommended to help reduce it. If you are overweight, you should be on a reducing diet. This reduced-calorie diet should be low in fat, no more than 30 percent. The fat you eat should include roughly equal amounts of saturated, polyunsaturated, and monounsaturated fat. Cholesterol intake should be no more than 300 milligrams daily. When you choose foods low in cholesterol, they usually are low in saturated fat too. Use the chart "Cholesterol in Foods" to tally up the content in the foods you eat.

If you follow this plan using the guidelines below, your cholesterol level will go down at least 10 to 15 percent:

CHOLESTEROL-LOWERING HINTS

1. Use liquid vegetable oils. Corn, soybean, sunflower, safflower, cottonseed (labeled VEGETABLE OIL)—in place of butter or solid fats. If you prefer olive oil for some purposes, it should be mixed with suggested oils (for example, ¼ cup olive oil plus ¾ cup corn oil equals 1 cup cooking oil).

2. Choose margarines with "liquid vegetable oil" as their first ingredient. When margarines are high in polyunsaturated fat they give this information on their label.

3. Limit beef, lamb, pork, or ham. These foods should be eaten only three times weekly. Use more fish, chicken, turkey, and veal. Shellfish, except shrimp, can be substituted for meat. Do not use liver or other organ meats. Use dried peas, beans, and lentils in place of meat two or more times weekly.

4. Use lean cuts of meat. Trim off all visible fat. Cook without added fat. Bake, broil, boil, or roast to further reduce fat.

5. Use skim milk and skim milk cheese and yogurt. No butter, cream, sour cream, or whole milk should be used.

6. Eat more fiber. Fiber reduces serum cholesterol levels. The fiber in unprocessed bran has no effect on cholesterol levels. Eat more vegetables and whole-grain cereals. Use fruits for snacks and desserts.

7. Limit eggs. Eat eggs only in cooked and baked foods. Reserve eggs as a main dish (omelets or poached) for occasional use, two or three times a month.

8. Avoid nondairy creamers and whipped toppings. Coffee whiteners and nondairy whipped toppings are high in saturated fat.

If you have a sweet tooth, you may indulge it occasionally with hard candies and jelly beans, which are free of fat, rather than chocolate, which contains saturated fat.

See the question "The doctor put my husband on a low-fat diet. . . ." for more suggestions that would be equally good on a low-cholesterol diet. Your diet should also emphasize polyunsaturated fat. See the following questions for suggestions on this.

CHOLESTEROL IN FOODS

Food	Portion	Milligrams of cholesterol	Calories
Margarine, vegetable oil	1 teaspoon	0	36
Bacon fat	1 tablespoon	1	126
Bread	1 slice	1	70
Milk, skim	1 cup	5	90
Sour cream	1 tablespoon	5	26
Cottage cheese, 1% fat	½ cup	5	81
Cream, half and half	1 tablespoon	6	20

Food	Portion	Milligrams of cholesterol	Calories
Chicken fat	1 tablespoon	9	126
Mayonnaise	1 tablespoon	10	100
Yogurt, low fat, fruit flavor	1 cup	10	231
Butter	1 teaspoon	11	36
Lard	1 tablespoon	12	126
Butter, unsalted	1 teaspoon	13	45
Fish sticks, frozen	1 stick	15	40
Sardines, canned in oil	1 sardine	15	40
Cottage cheese, creamed	½ cup	17	130
Caviar	1 tablespoon	25	32
Swiss cheese	1 ounce	26	104
Ice cream	½ cup	27	165
American cheese	1 ounce	27	93
Cheddar cheese	1 ounce	30	112
Milk, regular whole	1 cup	34	168
Cream cheese	2 tablespoons	34	99
Frankfurter	1	34	170
Cake, from mix with chocolate frosting	1 slice	36	175
Cinnamon roll	1	39	174
Salmon, broiled	3½ ounces	47	200
Clams	3½ ounces	50	52
Halibut, broiled	3½ ounces	60	214
Chicken, white meat	3 ounces	67	115
Beef	3 ounces	75	245
Chicken, dark meat	3 ounces	75	160
Veal, lean	3 ounces	85	210
Shrimp, fried	½ cup	120	225
Tuna, canned in oil	3½ ounces	125	197
Tuna, canned in water	3½ ounces	125	127
Shrimp, canned	3½ ounces	150	116
Egg	1 egg	252	78
Liver	3½ ounces	370	135
Chopped liver	3 ounces	735	210

HOW TO LOWER CHOLESTEROL IN YOUR MENU

TYPICAL DAY'S MENU	LOW-CHOLESTEROL MENU
Breakfast	
Grapefruit juice	Grapefruit
Poached egg	Cup cooked oatmeal with skim milk and teaspoon sugar
Buttered toast	Bran muffin with jelly
Coffee with cream	Coffee with skim milk
Lunch	
Tuna salad sandwich with lettuce	Tuna salad sandwich (use water-packed tuna and Special Dressing*)
Cole slaw	Green salad dressing with vinegar or lemon
Apple pie	Baked apple
Milk	Skim milk
Coffee with cream	Coffee with skim milk
Dinner	
Tomato juice	Tomato juice
Fried chicken	Broiled chicken
Mashed potatoes	Baked potato with yogurt topping
Carrots and peas	Carrots and peas
Jell-O with whipped cream	Banana or other fresh fruit
Tea with lemon	Tea with lemon
Snack	
Milk	Skim milk
Coffee cake	Graham crackers

* Special Dressing: 1 teaspoon mayonnaise plus 1 teaspoon plain yogurt.

* Why is polyunsaturated oil and margarine used in a low-cholesterol diet?

Fats are mixtures of different kinds of fatty acids—saturated, monounsaturated, and polyunsaturated. Fats that contain mainly saturated fatty acids, usually the type in meat,

			Milli-
		Milli-	grams
	Grams	grams	of
	of	of	choles-
	Calories	fat	sodium	terol

Egg Substitutes

	Calories	Grams of fat	Milligrams of sodium	Milligrams of cholesterol
Chono (General Mills)	39	1.0	95	0
Egg Beaters (Fleischmann's)	60	7.5	108	0
Eggstra (Tillie Lewis)	43	1.0	80	57
Scramblers (Morningstar Farms, Miles Laboratories)	57	3.0	150	0
Second Nature (Avoset Foods)	44	1.6	106	0
For comparison:				
Egg, medium	78	5.5	59	262

* Figures represent 1 serving, the equivalent of 1 fresh medium egg.

milk, butter, eggs, and cheese have been shown to increase serum cholesterol levels. While fats that are largely polyunsaturated, those in vegetable oils, nuts, and seeds are known to reduce serum cholesterol levels. That is why people on low-cholesterol diets are told to increase the amount of polyunsaturated fat they eat and at the same time reduce their intake of saturated fat. (See next question.)

There is still another type of fatty acid in the food you eat—monounsaturated. This type has no effect on serum cholesterol level. It does not help to lower cholesterol levels. Olive oil is very rich in monounsaturated fatty acid and that is why this popular oil is usually eliminated in low-cholesterol diets. Peanut oil is another vegetable oil that is high in monounsaturated fatty acid.

There is a wide variety of margarines available. Not all

are high in polyunsaturates. You must read the label to be sure that liquid oil is the first ingredient. If the first ingredient is hydrogenated vegetable oil, or partially hydrogenated vegetable oil, that margarine contains less polyunsaturated fat. Soft margarines sold in tubs or tubes are generally higher in polyunsaturates than the stick or cube types.

* I was told to increase the polyunsaturated fats I eat and decrease the saturated fat. What value is this and how can I do it?

It has been shown repeatedly that blood cholesterol levels fall when you eat less saturated fat and more polyunsaturated fat. As a rule, animal foods such as meat, milk, and cheese are high in saturated fats while plant foods like fruit, vegetables, cereals, and dried peas and beans are low. Additionally, plant foods are high in polyunsaturates. Vegetarians, who, by the nature of their diet, eat less saturated fat, have lower levels of blood cholesterol than the rest of us. Vegetarian diets also tend to be lower in calories and higher in fiber, which helps. Read more about this in Chapter 10.

Saturated fat is twice as potent in raising blood cholesterol as polyunsaturated fat is in lowering cholesterol. It would seem best then to eat foods that contain twice as much polyunsaturated fat as saturated. Very few foods fit that description: soft margarine, vegetable oils, freshwater fish, chicken, almonds, and walnuts. You can see that it would be hard to eat only these foods. What you can do is choose these in place of foods with small amounts of polyunsaturated fat like pork, beef, butter, and egg yolk whenever possible.

The following suggestions will help you to increase the ratio of polyunsaturates to saturates.

You can increase your intake of polyunsaturated fats and decrease saturated fats by eating more fruits, vegetables, dried peas and beans, and less food that comes from animals, such as meat and milk. You can eat practically any fruit or vegetable (coconut, chocolate, and thick-skinned avocados are exceptions), but you have to be more selective with the meat and dairy products you choose.

- Use skim milk and skim milk cheese and yogurt.
- Use poultry and fish in place of red meat. Small portions

(3 ounces) of beef, lamb, and pork can be eaten no more than two to three times a week.

• Use dried peas and beans, pasta with small amounts of cheese, and other nonmeat main dishes often. See Chapter 10 for suggestions about this.

• Eggs should be limited to three a week. Egg whites can be used as often as you like. Egg substitutes that are low in fat can be eaten. (See the chart "Egg Substitutes.")

• Don't use butter; it is high in saturated fat. Use margarines high in polyunsaturated fats. Generally, the softer types in tubs or tubes are more polyunsaturated than the stick types. Margarines that list liquid vegetable oil are the best to use. Choose margarines that give twice as much (or more) polyunsaturated fat as saturated fat. This will appear on the label; if it doesn't then it probably is not high in polyunsaturates.

• Use regular breads or home-baked biscuits, muffins, or other baked goods made with liquid vegetable oil. Many commercially available cakes, cookies, crackers, biscuit mixes, coffee cakes, Danish pastries, muffins, and other baked goods are made with saturated fats. This is so even if the label reads MADE WITH VEGETABLE SHORTENING because the shortening often used is from saturated vegetable oils—palm or coconut. You must read labels constantly as manufacturers often change their recipes—going from vegetable fat to lard for instance—as the price of lard becomes less.

• Use cereals, rice, macaroni, as you wish. Most noodles are made with eggs. Look for new products made with egg whites only (i.e., No Yolks Brand*).

• Use fruits, vegetables, and nuts except for coconut. Thick-skinned avocados are higher in saturated fat and should not be used. Use thin-skinned types.

• Other foods that can be used are coffee, coffee substitutes, tea, cocoa made with dry cocoa, skim milk (not chocolate-flavored), soft drinks, jams, jellies, maple syrup, honey, and molasses.

* Available from Foulds, Inc., Libertyville, Illinois.

* What are coffee whiteners? Can I use them on a low-cholesterol diet?

Even though their names may suggest cream, coffee whiteners, also called "nondairy creamers," do not contain cream. They are usually a mixture of vegetable fat (often palm oil or coconut oil), corn syrup, casein, and coloring, along with stabilizers and emulsifiers. One teaspoon of a typical powdered coffee creamer has 10 calories and little else in the way of nutrients.

These nondairy creamers should not be used if you are on a cholesterol-lowering diet because the fat they contain, palm or coconut oil, is a saturated fat even though it comes from a plant.

* On a low-cholesterol diet which oil is best for me to use?

Safflower oil is highest in polyunsaturates of all the usual cooking oils. However, it is not available in all stores and when it is, it's expensive. Corn, soybean, and cottonseed oil are high in polyunsaturates, and though not quite as rich a source as safflower oil, they are generally widely available and lower in cost. Sunflower oil is now available in many supermarkets and may be used. Cottonseed oil is often labeled just VEGETABLE OIL.

Peanut and olive oil are not as good sources of polyunsaturates and their use should be limited on a low-cholesterol diet. If you like the flavor of olive oil, try mixing it with one of the other more highly polyunsaturated oils (one-quarter cup olive oil plus three-quarters cup corn oil).

* Can I save oil in which I have fried foods to use over again?

It is not true that reusing oil for frying changes the oil from polyunsaturated to saturated. A study showed that heating corn oil seven times to 481°F (much higher than the temperature usually used for frying) caused no loss of linoleic acid. Linoleic acid is the main polyunsaturated fatty acid in corn oil. There is no reason to discard oil if you need to use it again once or twice. However, repeated reheating of oil to smoking changes its flavor and color, and this oil should be discarded.

* Will supplements of niacin reduce my cholesterol level?

Large amounts of niacin, 3 to 6 grams daily of the acid form of niacin, nicotinic acid (Nicobid, Nico-400) have been used to reduce serum cholesterol and other fat in the blood. In these amounts, however, the vitamin causes a rush of blood to the skin with a tingling, burning sensation especially on the face, neck, and hands. Another form of the vitamin, nicotinamide, does not cause this reaction but neither does it lower cholesterol levels.

Because of the flushing and other side effects (intestinal disturbances are one) niacin supplements are not commonly used to treat high serum cholesterol levels.

* Can green tea lower your cholesterol level?

Studies have shown that green tea can lower serum cholesterol in persons with higher than normal levels. Green tea is made from unfermented leaves, unlike the fermented black leaves we usually use for tea. Two cups of tea with lemon, sugar, and milk taken daily for fifteen days reduced cholesterol levels about 10 percent in people with levels over 250 milligrams.

* Will lowering my serum cholesterol level increase my risk of getting cancer?

Some studies have shown that people with low serum cholesterol levels seem more likely to get cancer, especially cancer of the colon. Reviewing the data raises the question— which came first, the cancer or the low serum cholesterol level? It has been suggested that undetected cancers may have reduced the cholesterol level in the people studied. In any case, the risk of cancer is increased very slightly and scientists have not been able to find a cause-and-effect relationship between cancer and low serum cholesterol levels. The more certain relationship is that between elevated cholesterol and heart attacks. It is wise to eat a diet low in cholesterol and fat and high in fiber to try to reduce your serum cholesterol level.

* What are the other risk factors for heart attack beside cholesterol?

Cigarette smoking is a significant risk and one that you can avoid. High blood pressure is another major risk and your pressure should be checked regularly. If it is persistently high, you need medical help and treatment. Salt restriction is usually part of the treatment and this will be covered elsewhere in this chapter. Weight loss, if you are overweight, is also needed. (Read about that in Chapter 7.)

Inactivity is another risk factor. If you haven't already done so, begin to plan for some regular exercise, even walking, for at least a half hour every other day. You'll feel better, use up some calories, and maybe reduce your risk of heart attack at the same time.

Some of us have competitive-type personalities, the type that is always impatient, rushing around, and overly ambitious. These people often do two things at one, like eating while driving the car. If you recognize yourself in this description, you should understand that this is coronary-prone behavior. Relaxation techniques and biofeedback may be useful to counteract these tendencies.

Other risk factors for heart attack that we can do little about are our age (as you get older, your risk is greater), your sex (men are at greater risk than women), diabetes, and a family history of heart disease.

HEART DISEASE

* Is atherosclerosis the same thing as hardening of the arteries?

Hardening of the arteries, also called *arteriosclerosis*, is a general term for the changes in arteries as we get older.

There is a thickening and loss of elasticity. *Atherosclerosis* refers to one part of the process—the depositing of fat on the inside walls of arteries. Eventually these deposits, also called "plaques," can block the flow of blood. When there is a partial blocking in the arteries leading to the heart, *angina*, a sudden severe pain in the chest (sometimes the left arm and shoulder too), develops during exercise or stress. If the artery is completely blocked, a heart attack results.

* Can homogenized milk cause heart attacks?

Some researchers believe that homogenization of milk, in which the fat globules are broken up and new particles of fat created, permits an enzyme in cow's milk BMXO (bovine milk xanthine oxidase) to damage blood vessel walls. BMXO is found in atherosclerotic plaques (see preceding question) and in the scar tissue of persons who have had heart attacks. It is not found in normal tissue. This theory, which attempts to pinpoint a cause of atherosclerosis, has been disputed by others. More research is needed before we will know what part, if any, homogenization of milk plays in the etiology of atherosclerosis.

* I have heard that HDL cholesterol is good. What is that?

Cholesterol is a fat and cannot dissolve into the blood, which is mainly water. Therefore, it travels along with protein as lipoproteins (fat plus protein). Low density lipoproteins (LDL) carry 50 to 75 percent of all blood cholesterol and high density lipoproteins (HDL) carry 15 to 25 percent.

The LDL cholesterol is believed to be excess that is deposited into the coronary arteries so that when LDLs are elevated there is a greater risk of atherosclerosis. On the other hand, HDL cholesterol is being carried to the liver, which excretes it. Therefore, a higher level of HDLs would be desirable. When you have higher levels of HDL you are less likely to get atherosclerosis and heart attack.

Premenopausal women, thin people, nonsmokers, people

who exercise regularly, and those who drink moderately tend to have higher levels of HDL.

You can increase your HDL levels by losing weight if you are overweight, following an exercise program, not smoking, and also drinking a moderate amount of alcohol. This means two mixed drinks (1½-ounce jiggers in each) or two 12-ounce cans of beer or two 5-ounce glasses of wine daily.

✳ I have heard that there is a pill coming out on the market soon that prevents heart attacks; where can I get it?

Perhaps you are referring to eicosapentaenoic acid (EPA). This is a type of lipid, a fat scientists have isolated from mackerel and other fish. This compound is found in large amounts in the food that Eskimos usually eat. The Eskimos' lifestyle is often studied, as they have a very low rate of heart disease. When volunteers ate large amounts of mackerel in addition to their regular food, their cholesterol and triglyceride levels went down considerably. They also had other changes in their blood that many doctors felt would put them at lower risk of heart attack. At the present time, there is no proof that EPA prevents heart attacks. There is not even evidence that EPA is not harmful. We look forward to more research over the next few years to help understand just how beneficial EPA may be. In the meantime, there would be no risk if you wish to increase the amount of EPA in your diet by eating more mackerel, salmon, anchovies, and cod.

✳ What is a cafe coronary?

A "cafe coronary" refers to choking on food. It has nothing to do with a heart attack, but the victim who is choking may be mistakenly thought to be having one. The symptoms of choking are similar to those of a heart attack. The person cannot breathe, becomes panicky, pale, and collapses. Immediate action is needed. Directions for the "Heimlich maneuver" are posted in many restaurants. The person who is giving aid stands behind the victim and places both arms around his or her chest just beneath the rib cage and hugs tightly in an effort to dislodge the food. We should all be familiar with the procedure for helping a choking victim.

HYPERTENSION

* What is hypertension?

People often think of high blood pressure as a "stress" disease resulting from tension. In fact, no one is sure what causes hypertension.

Hypertension, or high blood pressure, refers to a sustained rise in the pressure in the arteries. This pressure is actually the force of blood against the blood vessel walls. It is reported as two numbers written like this: 120/80. The upper figure, in this case 120, is the *systolic* pressure—the maximum pressure when the heart contracts and forces the blood through the arteries. The lower figure, in this case 80, is the *diastolic* pressure—the minimum pressure when the heart relaxes between beats. The normal range of blood pressure is about 100/60 to 120/80. Repeated measurements at or above 140/90 would be termed high blood pressure.

Nearly 60 million Americans are at risk of developing hypertension. About 24 million have it now, though many do not know it. By the time they are sixty-five, three out of four people are hypertensive. People with hypertension are more likely to get a heart attack, stroke, or kidney damage.

* What regulates blood pressure?

Our bodies regulate blood pressure by a combination of nerve signals and chemical responses that direct our arterioles to widen or narrow. *Arterioles* are small, muscular blood vessels that carry oxygen and nutrients from the larger arteries to the tissues. When part of the body needs nourishment, for example the stomach when we digest food, the arterioles surrounding the stomach expand, and arterioles in other areas of the body constrict. This balance maintains normal blood pressure. In the hypertensive person this system of balance doesn't work: arterioles constrict all over the body at the same time and stay constricted. This constriction causes the pressure in the larger arteries to go up and stay up—that is high blood pressure.

* How can I tell if I have hypertension?

You may have hypertension and not know it. It can cause damage for fifteen to twenty years before any symptoms appear. Some warning signs are headache, chest pains, shortness of breath, and heart palpitations, but you may not have any of these. All too frequently the first sign may be a heart attack or stroke, which can be fatal. That is why it is vital that everyone have his or her blood pressure checked *regularly*.

* My parents had high blood pressure. Will I have it also?

If your parents or other close relatives have high blood pressure, there is a good chance you will develop it too. Other people also at greater risk of being hypertensive are: males, females who are past menopause, younger women who take birth control pills, blacks, and those who are overweight.

You may wonder whether or not there is a hypertensive personality. Some people associate the term "hypertense" with being overly tense or anxious. It will interest you to learn that this personality type has been described variously as having "stressful personal interactions"; being "irritable, anxious, restless, and tense"; also as "dominant, assertive and decisive"; and as "emotionally more responsive, guarded, apprehensive." I guess most of us would fit in there somewhere and it follows that almost anyone can develop high blood pressure.

* Does salt cause high blood pressure?

The cause for high blood pressure in most people is not fully understood. Two nutritional factors are among several found to be associated with hypertension. One of these is salt intake, the other is obesity (discussed in Chapter 7). A relationship between salt intake and high blood pressure has been shown in studies done throughout the world. Those with high salt intake have more hypertension, while those who eat little or no salt do not. That is why it is felt that high blood pressure could be prevented in susceptible people if they ate less salt or, more precisely, less sodium. So while a cause-and-effect relationship between salt and hypertension has not been proven, there is strong support for limiting salt intake in those who are at risk. Those at risk are hard to identify, so it seems worthwhile to recommend a moderate reduction in salt intake for everyone. For people who have already been diagnosed as hypertensive, salt restriction along with weight control is often the initial treatment.

SALT AND SODIUM

* Is salt the same as sodium?

Many people confuse these two terms, even using them interchangeably. They are not the same. Salt, as it is used in a saltshaker, is a mixture of two minerals—sodium and chloride. If you took a teaspoon of salt, which weighs 5 grams, 2 of the 5 would be sodium and the other 3 grams would be chloride. Another way of saying that is that table salt is 40 percent sodium and 60 percent chloride.

When you are on a low-salt diet, sodium is the substance you are concerned with. Table salt is the most common source of sodium but there are many other sources too.

* I sometimes see sodium measured in milliequivalents (mEq) and other times as milligrams. What is the difference?

They are different units of measurement. To convert milliequivalents (mEq.) to milligrams (mg.) multiply the number of mEq. of the sodium by 23.

$$20 \text{ mEq. sodium} = 460 \text{ mg sodium}$$
$$20 \text{ mEq.} \times 23 = 460 \text{ mg of sodium}$$

To convert mg. to mEq. divide the number of mg. of sodium by 23.

$$506 \text{ mg. sodium} = 22 \text{ mEq.}$$
$$506/23 \text{ mg.} = 22 \text{ mEq. sodium}$$

The following chart will help you see the relationship between milligrams and milliequivalents of sodium and what they equal in salt.

SODIUM EQUIVALENTS

Milligrams of sodium	Millequivalents of sodium	Grams of salt
500	21.8	1.3
1,000	43.5	2.5
1,500	75.3	3.8
2,000	87.0	5.0

* Isn't some sodium necessary in my diet?

Yes, you do need sodium. There's some in every cell in your body (and in almost everything you eat too). It is estimated that adults need 200 to 500 milligrams a day. But most of us eat much more than we need—twenty or more times as much! Studies show that about one-third of this is from salt we sprinkle on food. The rest is there in the food itself, added in processing or added in cooking.

You can get all the sodium you need in a half-teaspoon of salt. You don't even need to add that much. If you ate an average daily diet of two cups of milk; 6 ounces of meat, fish, or poultry; four servings of bread and cereals; and four servings of fruit and vegetables, these foods would contain 500 milligrams of sodium naturally, even if no salt or other sodium-containing additives were used. It really isn't necessary for you to add salt to your food to get enough sodium.

* Which foods are naturally high in sodium?

Meat, fish, poultry, milk, cheese, and eggs are naturally high in sodium. These foods should be used in limited amounts if you are on a low-sodium diet. Organ meats and shellfish are higher in sodium than other meats and fish. You may be surprised to hear that saltwater fish like cod, mackerel, and striped bass do not contain more sodium than fish caught in freshwater (trout, whitefish).

Some vegetables like spinach, kale, carrots, artichokes, and celery have more sodium than other vegetables, but unless you are on a *very restricted* diet, you don't have to worry about this.

Fruits are very low in sodium and so are sugar, coffee, tea, jelly, oils, pasta, and unsalted butter or margarine. Cereals vary in sodium with cooked, lightly processed cereals like oatmeal being low and instant hot cereals and many cold cereals containing much more. Puffed wheat, puffed rice, and plain shredded wheat contain little sodium. Other cold cereals are high in sodium. However, Kellogg's and General Foods are reformulating their breakfast cereals to lower the sodium content. Check the labels to find out about your favorites. Cold cereals that are low in sodium can be found in health food stores and in the diet food section of your supermarket. Low-sodium cornflakes are the easiest to find. Bread, too, may be high in sodium: if you eat more than four or five slices daily, choose some low-salt types like matzoh. Many supermarkets carry at least one low-sodium bread. Ask the manager.

Even the water you drink can contain a lot of sodium. Check with your local health department to find out.

FOODS NATURALLY HIGH IN SODIUM

Artichokes	Greens	Milk
Celery	Spinach	Beets
Carrots	Egg white	White turnip

FOODS NATURALLY LOW IN SODIUM

Fruits	Shredded wheat	Rice
Coffee and tea	Puffed rice	Pasta
Jelly	Fresh fish	Oatmeal

SODIUM IN FOODS

Food	Milligrams of sodium	Portion
Corn, fresh	1	1 ear
Peanuts	1	4 tablespoons
Oatmeal, regular, cooked, no salt added	1	¾ cup
Pineapple, canned	1	1 slice
Butter, sweet	2	1 tablespoon
Coffee	2	6 ounces
Herb-Ox Low Sodium Beef broth*	9	1 packet
Celery, raw	25	1 stalk
Campbell's Low Sodium Corn soup*	30	10 ¾ ounces
Carrots, raw	34	1 medium
Saltine	35	1 cracker
Butter, salted	50	1 teaspoon
Chicken	57	3 ounces
Fudge	60	1 ounce
Egg	70	1 medium
Graham cracker	95	1 large
Peas, frozen	106	½ cup
Pepperidge Farm White bread	117	2 slices
Whole Milk	130	1 cup
Planters Cocktail Peanuts	132	1 ounce
White bread	140	1 slice
Heinz Tomato Ketchup	154	1 tablespoon
Skippy Creamy Peanut butter	167	2 tablespoons
Lay's Potato chips	191	1 ounce

* Many manufacturers are now marketing low-sodium versions of their products.

Food	Milligrams of sodium	Portion
Worcestershire sauce	206	1 table-spoon
Kraft American Cheese	238	1 slice (1 ounce)
Kellogg's Corn Flakes	260	1 ounce
Peanuts, salted	275	¼ cup
Taco Bell Bean Burrito	288	Entire serving
Campbell's Tomato juice	292	4 ounces
Oscar Mayer Bacon	302	3 slices
Wish-Bone Italian Salad dressing	315	1 table-spoon
Tomato juice	320	½ cup
Del Monte Sweet peas, canned	349	½ cup
Beef	381	3 ounces
Jell-O Chocolate Instant Pudding	404	½ cup
Devil's food pudding cake mix	435	1/12 of a cake
Frankfurter	495	1
English muffin, buttered	466	Entire muffin
Oscar Mayer Bologna	672	3 slices
Burger King Whaler	735	Entire serving
Herb-Ox Instant Broth, beef	818	1 packet
Burger King Whopper	909	Entire serving
Campbell's Beans & Franks	958	8 ounces
Heinz Dill pickles	1,137	1 large pickle
Swanson Fried Chicken Dinner	1,152	Complete dinner
Chef Boy-Ar-Dee Beefaroni	1,186	8 ounces
Soy sauce	1,320	1 table-spoon

Food	Milligrams of sodium	Portion
McDonald's Big Mac	1,510	Entire serving
Kentucky Fried Chicken Dinner, Extra Crispy	1,915	Dinner for 1 person
Kentucky Fried Chicken Dinner, Original Recipe Dinner	2,285	Dinner for 1 person

✳ What foods have had a lot of sodium added in processing?

This really includes many foods we all eat, even some unlikely ones, such as ice cream and instant pudding mixes. You really cannot always tell by taste alone. Some foods that taste and look salty (even when you can see the salt crystals on top) may actually contain less sodium than a sweet-tasting pastry or pudding. (See the chart "Sodium in Foods.")

Smoked, salted meats and fish including bacon, ham, corned beef, frankfurters, sausage, bologna, smoked salmon, dried codfish, finnan haddie, and others contain large amounts of sodium. So do pickles, olives, and sauerkraut that are packed in brine.

Canned fish and vegetables are packed in a salt solution and even some canned fruit has a little salt added to improve flavor and prevent darkening. Most frozen vegetables do not have added salt, except for peas and beans, which are sized in brine solutions. Frozen vegetables with added butter or sauces have more sodium than plain ones. Sauces and condiments such as ketchup, chili sauce, soy sauce, Worcestershire sauce, and even cooking wine contain lots of sodium.

If you want to know how much sodium is in a wide variety of foods, there was a useful booklet prepared in 1980 by the United States Department of Agriculture, "The Sodium Content of Your Food," Home and Garden Bulletin number 233. It is available from the Government Printing Office, Washington, D.C. 20402 (See also Appendix A.)

SODIUM-CONTAINING ADDITIVES

Additive	Use
Sodium saccharin	artificial sweetener
Monosodium glutamate (MSG)	seasoning, flavor enhancer, sold under brand names—Accent, Lawry's, McCormick
Sodium pyrophosphate	buffer and texturizer used in tuna and instant pudding mix
Sodium silicates	anticaking agent in salt
Sodium nitrite	preservative in cured meats
Sodium ascorbate	vitamin C
Sodium benzoate	preservative in soda, relishes, sauces, salad dressings
Sodium carboxymethyl cellulose	stabilizer in frozen desserts, salad dressings, chocolate milk
Sodium sulfite	used to bleach maraschino cherries or to preserve some dried fruits
Sodium hydroxide	used in processing of ripe olives, fruits, and vegetables to soften skins
Sodium propionate	mold inhibitor used in bread, cake, pasteurized cheese
Sodium erythorbate	preservative in processed meat such as hot dogs

* Are there any food additives that contain salt?

Many processed foods have sodium-containing additives. See chart above, "Sodium-Containing Additives." *Monosodium* glutamate (MSG) is a flavor enhancer. *Sodium* bicarbonate (baking soda) and *sodium* aluminum sulfate (baking powder) are used in bakery items. *Sodium* saccharin is an artificial sweetener. *Sodium* propionate inhibits mold in baked goods. *Sodium* sulfite is added to dried fruit to prevent discoloration. *Sodium* nitrite is in most luncheon meats, hot dogs, and bacon. Sodium may even be found in some carbonated beverages and mineral waters. (Perrier water is low in sodium.)

Here is the list of ingredients from a label for a common product many of us use. What do you think it is?

Corn syrup solids, partially hydrogenated vegetable oil (may contain one or more of the following oils: coconut, cottonseed, palm, palm kernel, or soybean), *sodium* caseinate, dipotassium phosphate, monoglycerides, *sodium* silicoaluminate, *sodium* tripolyphosphate, artificial flavors, beta carotene, and riboflavin.

These are the ingredients in a popular powdered nondairy coffee whitener. There are three sodium-containing additivies on the list. These should alert the person on a low-sodium diet to either avoid the food or limit its use. In this situation, because of the small amount of the whitener used in a serving, the sodium content, 5 milligrams in a teaspoon, is a negligible amount.

* Are there any other sources of sodium I should know about?

Yes, there are still other "hidden" sources of sodium you might not think about. Toothpaste often contains sodium as do many laxatives, antibiotics, cough medicines, antacids, and other drugs. (See the chart "Sodium in Antacids.")

Salt in the water you drink is often overlooked. The amount of this varies widely. Although "hard" water contains no more sodium than "soft" water, softening treatments often add sodium. Your local Department of Health can give you the sodium level in your water. Remember that the soda and beer you drink are bottled in varied locations. The sodium they contain will reflect the sodium level in the water used to make these beverages. The manufacturer can supply you with the sodium content of its beverage.

* How can I prepare tasty food without adding salt?

Many cookbooks are devoted to making a tasty food without added salt. (See the following question.) We have tried

SODIUM IN ANTACIDS

Antacid	Size	Milligrams of sodium
Alka-Seltzer	1 tablet	276.0
Amphojel	.3 gram tablet	1.4
	5 milliliters	6.9
Gaviscon	1 tablet	18.4
	5 milliliters	26.8
Lo-Sal	1 tablet	0.0
Maalox	1 #1 tablet	.84
	1 #2 tablet	1.80
	5 milliliters	2.5
Maalox Plus	1 tablet	1.4
Milk of magnesia	100 milliliters	10.0
Mylanta	1 tablet	5.0
	5 milliliters	5.0
Riopan	1 tablet	3.0
	5 milliliters	3.0
Riopan Plus	1 tablet	3.0
	5 milliliters	3.0
Rolaids	1 tablet	53.0
Sal Hepatica	1 dose	1,000.0
Sodium bicarbonate	1 dose	89.0
Tums	1 tablet	3.0

Note: 5 ml. = approximately a 1 teaspoon dose, 1000 ml. = 1 liter

liberal use of onion, garlic, lemon juice, and vinegar in salt-less recipes with great results. Other herbs and spices should be used less liberally or they may be overwhelming. A very light sprinkling of cayenne pepper will perk up a bland soup, while a larger amount could be painful. Because fresh spices and herbs are more flavorful than dried, use a little more of the fresh.

Use regular wine in cooking, not cooking wine, as this contains added salt. Unsalted bouillon cubes and unsalted tomato juice also make cooking without salt easier.

You can make your own saltless seasoning mix by combining your favorite herbs and spices. Try a saltless mixture we like.

Saltless Seasoning "Salt"

½ teaspoon garlic powder
¼ teaspoon powdered thyme
½ teaspoon onion powder
½ teaspoon paprika
¼ teaspoon ground celery seed
½ teaspoon pepper
½ teaspoon dry mustard

Mix together and store in a closed container in a dry place. Use this mixture as a general salt replacement on salads, meats, and vegetables.

* Is there a good cookbook I can get to help me make tasty foods without salt?

There are many good cookbooks and booklets available that can help you. One, now in its second edition, has a lot of useful information on reducing sodium and fat too—*The Fat and Sodium Control Cookbook* by Alma Payne and Dorothy Callahan, Little, Brown and Co., 1975.

Some other books for gourmets are:
Craig Claiborne's Gourmet Diet, Craig Claiborne with Pierre Franey, Ballantine Diet Cookbook, 1980.
Gourmet Cooking Without Salt, Eleanor Brenner, Doubleday, 1981.

Some paperbacks are:
Cooking Without a Grain of Salt, Elma W. Bogg, Bantam, 1964.
Cooking Without Your Salt Shaker, American Heart Association National Center, 7320 Greenville Avenue, Dallas, Texas 75231 1979 (or contact your local Heart Association).

A free booklet, "Delicious Low-Sodium Diets," is available from Standard Brands, Inc., 625 Madison Avenue, New York, New York 10022.

* I am on a low-salt diet and I like to make biscuits. What can I substitute for baking powder, which is high in sodium?

You can buy low-sodium baking powder in health food stores and supermarkets. You can also make your own:

Low-Sodium Baking Powder

1 tablespoon potassium bicarbonate (buy at the drugstore)
2 tablespoons cream of tartar
2 tablespoons arrowroot powder

Combine all ingredients thoroughly; store in an airtight container. Stir before you measure.

This baking powder may be used as an equivalent to regular baking powder in your recipes. Do remember to stir it before measuring because the powder tends to separate upon standing.

* Is a low-sodium diet the same as a salt-free diet?

No, the so-called salt-free diet usually means that no table salt is added to foods. This is sometimes called the "no salt-shaker diet." For a low-sodium diet, you need to think about the natural sodium in the foods as well as the salt used in processing, not just the salt added at the table.

* How can I stick to a low-salt diet when I eat in a restaurant?

When eating out, either in a fast food or regular restaurant, you can select those foods that contain the least added salt or sodium. Choose fruit or fruit juice for a first course instead of soup. (Tomato juice comes with much added salt. Don't order it.) If you want to nibble while waiting for your food, try plain bread, raw vegetables, or unsalted crackers (no dip). Mixed salads are fine, but add your own dressing, which can be a squeeze of lemon or a little vinegar and some oil. You may enjoy pepper to point up the flavor of the greens. The waitress will supply you with any of these, if you ask.

Ask for plain vegetables—no sauce, no salt. Baked potatoes are fine. Season them with a *little* sour cream instead of the salted butter that is usually available. (Chives are good.) Some restaurants may serve unsalted (sweet) butter. Ask for it and enjoy it if it is available. You will be surprised to see how good a baked potato tastes with no topping at all. Try it.

Plain broiled or baked fish, poultry, or meat usually is made with less salt than are mixtures of meat and vegetables with rice or pasta. If you wish a mixed dish, ask for the sauce or gravy on the side, then you can add only a tiny bit. For dessert, try fresh fruit, a baked apple, sponge or angel cake. The fruit salad or melon offered as an appetizer makes a fine dessert.

In a fast food restaurant, ask for the hamburger or fried fish without the sauce, ketchup, mayonnaise, or pickle. You can enjoy french fries; just ask for your portion without salt. You may have to wait until the next batch is fried so they can serve your portion before sprinkling on the salt.

In Chinese restaurants you can ask the waiter to have your portion prepared without added salt, soy sauce, or MSG. The waiter won't bat an eyelid! Steak and seafood restaurants will also prepare your meal to order—without added salt.

You can enjoy a cocktail, wine, coffee, tea, milk, or fruit juice with your meal. Stay away from Bloody Marys: they have tomato juice as well as Worcestershire sauce—too high in sodium.

* I am on a low-salt diet. Is sea salt better for me than regular salt?

They are practically the same. Both must contain at least 97.5 percent sodium chloride to be labeled salt, and therefore both are extremely high sources of sodium. If you are on a low-salt diet, you must limit both regular salt and sea salt.

Sea salt has often been touted as a good source of iodine. Actually most of the iodine is lost as the salt is evaporated from the seawater. Sea salt is essentially the same as regular salt and it's not worth paying extra for it.

* Do I have to add salt to the water I use to boil spaghetti and rice?

Label directions on pasta, noodles, and rice often direct cooking in boiling, salted water. Adding this salt is not necessary for proper cooking, it is suggested simply because of taste. The same is true of the directions on frozen vegetable packages. When you add salt to the cooking water, you are adding it unnecessarily.

* Should I take salt tablets when I exercise in hot weather?

The usual rule of thumb for taking extra salt when you exercise in the heat is that if you lose four quarts of water via sweating in one day, you need 1 more gram of salt. That's one-fifth of a teaspoon or the amount in one salt tablet. In most situations it isn't necessary nor is it desirable to take a salt tablet. A better approach is to drink plenty of water, diluted fruit juice, lemonade, orangeade, or a sports drink like Gatorade. Most athletes dilute sports drinks with an equal amount of water to reduce their concentration. This is a good idea.

Routine exercise—a jog, a game of golf, or a bike ride—does not call for salt tablets.

* I like salty foods. Does that mean I need salt?

You have learned to like salty foods because you probably have eaten salty foods all your life. In areas of the world where people have not been exposed to salty food, they do not wish for it. Research studies show that babies will just as readily eat unsalted food as salted. In fact, small children will choose unsalted food over salted.

If you have learned to prefer salty tastes, you can also unlearn this preference. By gradually reducing the salt you add in cooking and at the table you will become accustomed to the new flavor of unsalted foods. Eating becomes more of a pleasure as you can taste the subtle flavors of food that had been masked by salting. We have found that almost without exception added salt is not needed for delicious tasting foods. After you become accustomed to enjoying foods with less salt or no salt added, highly salted foods will taste far too salty to be enjoyed. If you smoke or drink a lot of coffee, you probably salt your food liberally, as both these practices tend to mask the flavor of food.

* I use kosher meat. How can I reduce the sodium content?

Meat is salted in the koshering process so that koshered meat contains much more sodium, approximately 330 to 380 milligrams in a 3-ounce portion. This is an extremely high amount for someone on a sodium-restricted diet. The sodium can be reduced by first salting the meat slightly and allowing it to stand for the prescribed time, then rinsing the meat and soaking it in water. After these two steps have been completed, the meat is boiled in a large quantity of water and the resulting broth is discarded. The drawback to this method is obvious; the meat will become tasteless and can be tough. However, the sodium content has been reduced to approximately 65 milligrams in 3 ounces. After reducing the sodium content by this method, skillful use of herbs can make the

---

HOW TO BREAK THE SALT HABIT

Empty your salt shaker and don't refill it.

Reduce or eliminate salt used in cooking. Don't add salt when cooking rice, pasta, or vegetables; it is not needed.

Limit the use of processed foods, especially "convenience" foods like TV dinners, pot pies, canned soups, gravies, sauces, and seasoned rice mixes.

Substitute low-salt snacks like fresh fruit; vegetable sticks; unsalted nuts, pretzels, or popcorn for the usual salty nibbles.

Stay away from salt-preserved foods like bacon, bologna, anchovies, sardines, pickles, sauerkraut, and olives.

Watch out for salty condiments like soy sauce, ketchup, Worcestershire sauce. Use lemon, vinegar, herbs, spices (not garlic, onion, and celery salt) instead.

In restaurants, ask them not to salt or use MSG when food is prepared.

Use low-salt cheeses, canned tuna, peanut butter, and unsalted margarine and sweet butter.

meat more tasty. If you are on a salt-restricted diet, contact your local rabbi for special permission to broil meat without koshering it first.

A person who observes the Jewish dietary laws has special problems on a low-sodium diet. In addition to the salting of meats during the koshering process, many other foods are extremely salty. The most common salted foods are lox, whitefish, corned beef, pastrami, tongue, cucumber pickles, pickled green tomatoes, pickled peppers, and sauerkraut. These foods are exceptionally high in salt and may have to be eliminated completely.

* Does potassium protect against the harmful effects of sodium for people with high blood pressure?

Evidence is accumulating that the ratio of sodium to potassium may be more important than the level of sodium alone. It is possible that both high-sodium and low-potassium intake is needed to set the stage for high blood pressure.

Processed foods tend to have potassium leached out in processing, and sodium added. It may be that eating mainly processed foods contributes to high blood pressure more than just a high sodium intake. Because this idea is still being studied, it would be unwise to dose yourself with potassium in an effort to avoid or to treat high blood pressure. Excess accumulation of potassium can be dangerous since it will disturb the body's mineral balance.

* How is Lite Salt different from salt substitutes?

Salt substitutes like Lite Salt (Morton) is half sodium chloride and half potassium chloride. One teaspoon contains 975 milligrams sodium compared to 2,300 milligrams sodium in a teaspoon of regular salt. This should not be confused with salt substitutes (Adolph's, Co-Salt, Diamond Feather-weight, Morton) that have less than 10 milligrams of sodium in a teaspoon and are used for sodium-restricted diets. Using Lite Salt is a way to reduce sodium intake and still use the salt shaker.

* Are potassium-containing salt substitutes a good source of potassium if I am on a diuretic?

Yes, they are. One teaspoon of a popular brand, Adolph's, contains 2,378 milligrams of potassium. Diamond and Morton contain about 2,500 milligrams. Check the label of the type you wish to use and then check with your doctor. Most people can safely use these salt substitutes and they have been shown to be an excellent source of the potassium that is lost when you use some diuretics.

Caution: Lite Salt, which is half regular sodium and half potassium, is not the same product. This may not be good for you if you are on a low-sodium diet. Again, check with your doctor before using any salt substitute.

* If I am on a diuretic, can I get all the potassium I need from foods instead of a supplement?

Many people take diuretics like Lasix (furosemide) and Diuril (chlorothiazide) that cause a loss of potassium as well as salt and water (not all diuretics cause this loss). Also combination drugs used to treat high blood pressure often contain a diuretic. In most cases, you can replace the potassium lost by using pleasant potassium-rich foods instead of taking a supplement, which is bitter tasting. You don't even need to increase your food (or calorie) intake. Some easy food substitutions will be sufficient.

Use whole-wheat bread in place of white bread. Boiling food causes potassium loss in the water. Use baked or steamed foods to retain most of the potassium. Eat a baked potato instead of boiled. Fresh fruit is better than canned unless you eat all the syrup. Oranges and bananas have a well-deserved reputation for being high in potassium. One of each will give you 900 milligrams of potassium. (This is the amount often contained in a maintenance dose of a potassium supplement.) A tomato is another good source. See the chart "Sodium and Potassium in Foods" for other high potassium choices that are also low in sodium.

Ask your doctor about using the potassium chloride salt substitutes. It can be an additional, inexpensive potassium source.

Sodium and Potassium in Foods

Food	Portion	Milligrams of sodium	Milligrams of potassium	Calories
Kidney beans, red	½ cup	10	984	343
Hamburger	4 ounces	82	960	280
Avocado	½	6	924	196
Sunflower seed kernels	3½ ounces	30	920	560
French fries	3½ ounces	4	652	220
Potato, baked no skin	1	4	503	95
Liver, calf	3½ ounces	118	453	261
Veal cutlet	3½ ounces	46	448	194
Pork chop	1 (3 oz.)	41	386	170
Milk, low fat	1 cup	122	381	102
Banana	1 small	1	370	85
Milk, whole	1 cup	120	370	150
Orange-grapefruit juice, canned	1 cup	3	335	95
Leg of lamb	2 ounces	52	312	107
Orange	1 medium	2	300	73
Sweet potato	1 medium	12	300	141
Pineapple juice	¾ cup	2	284	104
Chicken broiled	3½ ounces	66	274	136
Broccoli	1 stalk	10	267	26
Artichoke hearts	3½ ounces	47	248	26
Tomato, raw	1 small	3	244	22
Fried chicken	¼ bird	80	242	232
Corn, fresh	1 ear	Trace	196	100
Mango	½ medium	7	189	66

Sodium and Potassium in Foods (*cont.*)

Food	Portion	Milli-grams of sodium	Milli-grams of potassium	Calories
Orange juice, frozen	⅖ cup	1	186	45
Roast beef	2 thin slices (2 oz.)	17	169	70
Apple	1 medium	1	165	87
Bean sprouts	1 cup	4	156	28
Oatmeal	1 cup	1	130	148
Pear	1 medium	2	130	61
Blueberries	1 cup	1	113	81
Peanuts, roasted	1 tablespoon	Trace	111	86
Orange drink, instant	1 cup	16	108	143
Almonds, unsalted	12 to 15	Trace	104	90
Green beans	½ cup	3	95	16
Bread, whole-wheat	1 slice	121	63	56

✳ Is it true that asparagus acts like a diuretic?

People often think that some vegetables, particularly asparagus, act as diuretics, increasing the amount of urine. That's probably because after you eat asparagus, you can detect its odor in your urine. But asparagus has no diuretic effect nor does any other vegetable. Coffee and tea, because of their caffeine content, do cause increased urination. Other caffeine-containing products have the same effect. (See the chart "Sources of Caffeine" in Chapter 4.) Alcohol also is a diuretic and promotes loss of fluid from the body.

SPECIAL SALAD DRESSINGS

* I like my salad with dressing. Are there any that are low in salt and fat?

Yes, the classic low-salt, low-fat, low-cholesterol dressing is called, appropriately "Zero Dressing." Here is the recipe:

Zero Dressing
Makes approximately 1½ cups

1 cup low-sodium tomato juice
¼ cup lemon juice
2 tablespoons chopped onion
⅛ teaspoon pepper
1 teaspoon chopped fresh parsley, or
  ¼ teaspoon dry parsley
1 clove garlic, finely minced
2 tablespoons chopped pepper (optional)
¼ teaspoon dry mustard (optional)

Combine all ingredients in a screwtop jar; shake to blend. Store in refrigerator.

2 tablespoons contains 6 calories, 1 mg. sodium, 0 g. fat, and 0 mg. cholesterol

If you would rather use regular canned tomato juice, two tablespoons of Zero Dressing would have 6 calories, 60 mg. sodium, 0 g. fat, and 0 mg. cholesterol.

Following are a few more salad dressings you might like to try. Note that Creamy Green Dressing and Blue Cheese Dressing are higher in fat than Zero Dressing and Honey Dressing. However, they still are lower than most commercial salad dressings. For example, two tablespoons of bottled Roquefort dressing has 142 calories, 206 mg. sodium, and 14.6 g. fat.

Honey Dressing
Makes approximately 1¼ cups

1 cup low-fat plain yogurt
3 tablespoons orange juice
1 tablespoon lemon jucie
1 tablespoon honey

Combine all ingredients thoroughly and store in refrigerator in a covered container.

NOTE: This dressing is especially good on fresh fruit or over cottage cheese. Try it on freshly grated carrots for a unique vegetable slaw.

2 tablespoons: 30 calories, 20 mg. sodium, .4 g. fat, and 1.8 mg. cholesterol

Creamy Green Dressing
Makes approximately 1¼ cups

1½ cups cooked broccoli flowerets
½ cup plain low-fat yogurt
2 tablespoons vegetable oil
2 tablespoons lemon juice
1 garlic clove, crushed
Dash of cumin

Combine all ingredients in a blender container; process until smooth.

Store in the refrigerator in a covered container.

2 tablespoons: 50 calories, 13 mg. sodium, 3.8 g. fat, and .8 mg. cholesterol

Blue Cheese Dressing
Makes approximately ¾ cup

2 ounces blue cheese
⅔ cup low-fat plain yogurt
2 tablespoons lemon juice or vinegar
⅛ teaspoon dill weed
Pinch of garlic
Pinch of pepper

Crumble blue cheese and combine with remaining ingredients.

Store in refrigerator in a covered container.

2 tablespoons: 50 calories, 140 mg. sodium, 2.8 g. fat, and 7.8 mg. cholesterol

9

Living Longer

How long you live and how vigorously you live is something over which you have control. We frequently believe that our life is predetermined by our genetic code. This is simply not so. A good gene package is advantageous, but even if both of your parents are long-living this will add only three years to your average life-span and can be quickly wiped out by abuse. As we age, our susceptibility to disease, aches, and pains increases. Between thirty-five and forty-four cancer risks increase, with heart disease taking its toll after forty-five. These risks double after age fifty-five and by sixty-five the risk of stroke increases dramatically. All risks climb steadily through age eighty-five.

What control do you have over these? We know aging is inevitable and in fact begins at birth. We'd like to stress the enjoyment of a vigorous, long, and healthy life. This can be achieved by taking control of those risks you can manipulate, namely stress, exercise, and nutrition. Good health habits can add ten to fifteen years to our average life-span of seventy-three, allowing us to live in good health till approximately ninety.

We often read stories about extreme longevity, but careful investigation has found that most centarians are in truth younger than they claim. The oldest documented person is one-hundred-sixteen. There is, however, a special group of people who do live in good health to ninety-plus. What are their secrets? They appear quite simple—but in practice few people will find them easy to adhere to on a day-to-day basis.

241

Topping the longevity agenda is exercise, which is aerobic—walking, dancing, and cycling. The amount of exercise conducive to long life is the equivalent of walking ten miles a day. Soviet Georgians and other very old people exercise as part of their daily routine, during both work and recreation.

The second key to long life is a low-calorie intake with limited amounts of fat, sugar, and salt. Most of those people who are ninety-plus state a preference for nonmeat foods though few are vegetarians. This preference provides a nutrition bonus since grains, fruit, and vegetables are high in fiber, vitamins, and minerals while at the same time low in fat. Low calories plus exercise results in a lean body type, typical of most who have lived past ninety.

The last and very crucial key to longevity is personality. A profile of the ideal to strive for would be a person who has a strong self-image, successfully manages stress, and paces himself or herself so that he or she never reaches the point of exhaustion.

These suggestions should allow you to remain healthy from forty to sixty and continue from sixty to eighty in the same good health you experienced before. It's tempting to try shortcuts—unproven disease cures, vitamin and mineral supplements, fad diets—which do not force you to make changes in your lifestyle. Most of these will give little or no improvement in your health and well-being and, in some instances, may cause harm.

Good health and long life do not just happen. It takes a day-to-day conscious effort to manipulate risks to your advantage. In this chapter we will discuss ways to deal with problems we all face as we get older. We can manage most of these conditions so that our health and lifestyle remain vigorous and enjoyable.

* Can good nutrition guarantee me freedom from disease?

Risk factors are associated with good health and long life. Increase your risks and you increase the probability of getting certain diseases—high blood pressure, heart attack, cancer, and diabetes, among others. Decrease your risks and you can lengthen your life and enhance its quality.

Diet is a risk factor. It is not a miracle cure, panacea, or guarantee of longevity. But sound nutrition based on moderation, balance, and variety—in short, what we've been suggesting throughout this book—can reduce your risk of disease and add years to your life.

Seven health-related behavior patterns have been identified that reduce disease and protect against premature death. They are simple, and anyone could easily follow these patterns to insure better health and a longer life. Unfortunately, few do. Below are the seven positive health behaviors. How many do you practice?

1. Limit alcohol consumption to one or two drinks a day.
2. Eat three meals a day without snacking between.
3. Eat breakfast.
4. Maintain a normal weight.
5. Do regular physical exercise.
6. Sleep seven or eight hours a night.
7. Don't smoke cigarettes.

Four of these behaviors are related to nutrition. If a forty-five-year-old man followed three or four of these practices, he could expect to live to sixty-seven. Following all seven, his average life-span increases to seventy-eight.

ARTHRITIS

* What is arthritis?

Arthritis is a general term for over one hundred different ailments affecting over 31 million Americans. Osteoarthritis, the most common kind of arthritis, develops because of wear and tear on the joints, from overuse, stress, or injury. You are more likely to have osteoarthritis as you get older. It is usually mild.

Rheumatoid arthritis is the most serious type and can lead to crippling. It tends to have periodic flare-ups and can spread throughout the body, affecting joints and vital organs. Because the nature of this disease is that it comes and goes, the sufferer may believe that he or she is getting relief because of some "treatment" he or she is using. This makes the sufferer easy prey for quack cures.

* Is arthritis an autoimmune disease?

The immune system is a very complex network of cells and proteins, called "antibodies," that help to protect the body from infection and help to repair it when it is injured. When an infection develops, special immune cells recognize that a foreign substance—a bacteria or virus—is in the body, and then an elaborate series of events is started. Certain cells make antibodies directed against the infection and, with the help of other specialized cells, destroy the organisms responsible for the infection. Likewise, if a splinter is not removed from your finger, the tissue around it becomes reddened and painful. That shows that your body is trying to destroy the foreign material.

In certain situations, for reasons that are not understood, the immune system may direct antibody and specialized cells against normal parts of the body. This results in *autoimmune disease*—disease which involves the immune system fighting its own body. Rheumatoid arthritis is an example of an autoimmune disease. We do not know why or how these diseases occur (much research is currently under way to answer these questions) but we do know that by giving drugs that interfere with some aspects of the immune system, the symptoms of these diseases may be improved. Not all types of arthritis are due to autoimmune disease, but rheumatoid arthritis is.

* Could you tell me anything more about the foods that "cure" arthritis?

Ruth Stout, at eighty-eight, suggested a cure for arthritis. Eat brewer's yeast, bananas, wheat germ, pecans, and avocados. Miss Stout claims that ten days after being on this diet (she didn't always eat the avocados because they were too expensive!), her arthritis was gone, and it hasn't come back. She went on to *cure* her postman and counsels and advises all who question her about the diet. The five foods need not be eaten exclusively nor in any systematic fashion.

Is the diet a hoax or a help? This can't be answered because Miss Stout's experience is anecdotal, or observational.

No clinical tests have been run and no data analyzed. Eating brewer's yeast, bananas, wheat germ, pecans, and avocados (if they're not too expensive) along with other foods will not hurt an arthritis sufferer. This remedy is reasonably harmless. Others are not and may cause further suffering. As we've stressed before, be wary of miraculous cures and wonder treatments. They usually do not turn out to be that wonderful.

* Can diet cure arthritis?

Of all the questions we are asked, this is one of the most frequent. And we truly wish we had a good answer, a diet prescription that could cure arthritis. As with any chronic condition, good nutrition will help but by itself it is not a cure.

Diet remedies are suggested all the time. Dan Dale Alexander wrote *Arthritis and Common Sense* over thirty years ago and it is still selling today. Alexander recommends eating large amounts of oil, which will find its way to the joints and lubricate them. Physiologically this is impossible. Dietary oil would not remain intact after its journey through the digestive tract. This remedy surely does not help arthritis and the added oils may increase risks for heart disease, cancer, gallstones, and obesity.

Other cures suggested are apple cider vinegar, rutin, and blackstrap molasses (see Chapter 3), lecithin, alfalfa, yucca extract, and a starvation diet. Nothing eaten will cause arthritis inflammation or cure it.

Good eating habits and plenty of calcium are good advice for the arthritic sufferer. The chronic pain may cause a loss of appetite, and morning stiffness makes preparing breakfast a chore. It that's the case, eat a mid-morning snack to make up for the small breakfast and eat your main meal midday when you have the least pain. Drugs prescribed often interfere with nutrients. Aspirin destroys vitamin C, so extra food sources or a supplement are needed. (See Chapter 4 for more information on drug-nutrient interaction.)

Vitamin E supplements have been suggested for osteoarthritis. Daily supplements of 600 milligrams gave "marked improvement" in ten days to a small group of people. Further study may show that vitamin E can offer pain relief to the arthritis sufferer.

* Can I find relief from my arthritis if I stop eating nightshade vegetables?

Our educated guess would be no. This question, however, is one we cannot answer definitely. And believe us, we've tried!

Nightshades include herbs, shrubs, and plants of the genus *Solanum.* Vegetables in this group are the white potato, tomato, eggplant, pepper, and apples. Excluding these foods from the arthritic's diet is supposed to eliminate pain and inflammation. Testimonials claim that it works. Authorities can find no scientific link between these foods and arthritis. One theory, yet unproven, is that some arthritic sufferers may be allergic to these foods and the allergic reaction is what causes joint pain and inflammation.

Arthritis is a chronic and complicated disorder whose normal course often results in periods of little discomfort. It is difficult to tell how much relief is gained from home remedies. More than 30 million people have arthritis. Even when under medical treatment, about 60 percent simultaneously try home remedies—alfalfa seeds, sea brine, vitamin and mineral supplements, and liniments. It's been estimated that $950 million a year is spent on unproven remedies. Your nearest chapter of the Arthritis Foundation can often help sort out fact from fallacy. Check your phone book or write to the national office at 3400 Peachtree Road N.E., Atlanta, Georgia 30326.

For more information, the Arthritis Foundation recommends in its "Guide to Books on Arthritis" that the following books have reliable information about arthritis. It warns: "Some books on arthritis are patently misleading and contain statements that simply are not true, according to the best medical knowledge today. Such books are not recommended. . . ."

Arthritis, A Comprehensive Guide, James F. Fries, M.D., Addison-Wesley Publishing Co., 1979.

The Arthritis Helpbook—What You Can Do for Your Arthritis, Kate Lorig, R.N., James F. Fries, M.D., Addison-ley Publishing Co., 1980.

Beyond the Copper Bracelet—What You Should Know about Arthritis, 2nd ed., Louis A. Healey, M.D., Kenneth R. Wilske, M.D., Bob Hansen, Charles Press Publishers, 1977.

Overcoming Arthritis, Frank D. Hart, M.D., Arco Publishing, 1981.

Wellness: An Arthritis Reality, Beth Ziebell, Ph.D., Kendall/Hunt Publishing Co., 1981.

* I'm an arthritis sufferer and a friend warned me not to eat licorice. Why?

Your friend is right to a certain degree. Natural licorice extract used to flavor imported licorice candy may affect the action of anti-inflammatory drugs used to relieve arthritis pain. Licorice candy and flavoring used in the United States is artificial and not made from natural licorice extract. If you are taking a drug such as Butazolidin, Clinoril, Tolectin, or Motrin, you should not eat imported licorice candy.

Imported licorice may interfere with the action of diuretics such as Aldactone, HydroDiuril, Oretic, and Lasix.

* Will DMSO help my arthritis?

When you have arthritis and are in chronic pain, any remedy, no matter how controversial, is inviting. Breakthroughs in treatment, real or not, get wide publicity on radio, television, and in magazines. Sensational headlines suggest "cures" or at the least "relief." DMSO, an alleged breakthrough, is currently attracting attention. Dimethylsulfoxide (DMSO) is used only as a veterinary drug. Nevertheless, zealous support for its use as an arthritis treatment has gotten state approval in Florida and Oregon. The government does not allow it to be used in humans, except in an injectable form for a bladder disorder. In studies with an arthritic skin disease (scleroderma) DMSO was not helpful. Although used often to treat arthritis, its effectiveness has never been established and it has dangerous side effects, such as chemical burns and damage to vision. We'd urge caution if you were considering self-treatment with DMSO.

* Is it true that eating mussels will eliminate my arthritis pain?

You can add mussels to the ever-growing list of worthless arthritis remedies. The product being promoted is actually the extract of New Zealand green-lipped mussels sold in health food stores as Seatone, Freedom, or Aquatone. Promotions claim the extract will relieve both rheumatoid and osteoarthritis. These claims, as with others, are based on dramatic personal testimony and research published in a lesser-known medical journal of questionable authority. The Arthritis Foundation has refuted the remedy as unfounded and cautioned that the mussel extract has not been shown to be safe. Unfortunately, unless the Food and Drug Adminstration can bar the import of the mussel extract, millions will probably buy it looking for relief.

GOUT

* What is gout?

Gout can be considered a birth defect (an inborn error of metabolism) that doesn't show up till we're adults. Men, who have gout more frequently than women, show signs of the problem around thirty-five. For the rare woman with gout, her problem will not begin till after menopause.

A gout sufferer cannot efficiently eliminate uric acid from his body. It builds up and deposits form in small joints and surrounding tissue. The toes, particularly the large toe, becomes painful and the pain may radiate up the leg. If it is diagnosed (a simple blood test can usually detect gout) and treated with medication, most gout sufferers find the problem is mild and only occasionally causes discomfort. (See the following question for more information.)

* Is gout caused by eating too many rich foods?

The typical picture of a gout sufferer is the stout old gentleman, sitting amidst splendor with his foot propped on a satin pillow. The scene suggests that lavish living leads to gout. As we discussed in the preceding question, gout is an error of metabolism that a person inherits. It is not caused by food or alcohol, though both have been implicated. Even so, some diet considerations can help the gout sufferer keep the condition mild.

Today, drugs are used to regulate uric acid, so dietary treatment is less important. However, a diet high in carbohydrate, low in fat, and moderate in protein will aid the drug's action controlling the uric acid level. Carbohydrate foods tend to increase uric acid elimination, so the gout sufferer should rely heavily on breads, cereals, vegetables, and fruit. A high-fat intake—butter, salad dressing, fried foods—slows down uric acid elimination and may induce a gouty attack in some people. Overeating, fasting, use of water pills, as well as being overweight are all conditions that aggravate gout and will cause more frequent painful episodes.

Certain foods, when they are broken down in the body, yield substantial amounts of uric acid. It is wise to limit their use and to exclude them from the diet altogether during painful periods. These foods are listed in the highlight box "Bothered with Gout?"

Gout sufferers are often told not to drink alcohol, coffee, tea, or cocoa. Although alcohol does not cause gout, it interferes with the elimination of uric acid. An occasional drink is fine, but overindulgence is unwise. Coffee, tea, and cocoa are broken down to methylurates, but this substance is not deposited in joints as is uric acid. Thus they need not be avoided. (See the following box for many suggestions that are helpful in preventing gouty attacks.)

For relief during painful attacks, limit protein intake to 3 ounces a day and use only vegetable and dairy proteins like

---

BOTHERED WITH GOUT?

<u>Do</u>
maintain ideal weight.
eat large amounts of
  carbohydrate foods.
eat moderate amounts of
  protein foods.
drink eight to ten glasses of
  liquid a day.

<u>Don't</u>
overeat.
fast.

use large amounts of alcohol.

eat large amounts of fatty
  foods.
eat anchovies, gravies, broth,
  liver, herring, mincemeat,
  mussels, scallops, brewer's
  yeast.

---

beans, cheese, and yogurt. At the same time, cut out fat and drink three or more quarts (twelve cups) of fluid a day to help clear the body of the uric acid buildup.

ULCERS

* Does excessive stomach acid cause ulcers?

The idea that stomach acid causes ulcers is widely held. It is false. Once an ulcer is formed, stomach acid may irritate and worsen the condition but the acid did not cause it. In a healthy person, the stomach lining is well protected by mucus and the natural acidity should not cause damage.

Ulcers appear to be due to a weakness in the intestinal wall. Why some have this weak spot is unknown. Poor nutrition, lack of rest, or a genetic flaw have all been suggested. Excessive anxiety and worry may be a cause: "It is not what he eats, it's what is eating him . . ."

Regardless of the cause, excessive acid secretion, provoked by stress and anxiety will rapidly make the ulcer worse. Learning to relax and cope with the stress of life may be the best treatment for the ulcer sufferer.

* Is there more than one kind of ulcer?

Yes, there is. Duodenal ulcers, the most common, are found in the beginning of the small intestine. Gastric ulcers are in the stomach. Both are called peptic ulcers and occur in men more often than in women.

An ulcer results when the top layer of cells in the wall of the stomach or duodenum are eroded, leaving underlying cells exposed. These delicate cells are painful when touched by stomach contents and will continue to wear away until bleeding or perforation (a hole) results. (See the following questions for more information about causes and treatment of ulcers.)

* I have an ulcer, but my doctor did not give me a strict diet to follow. Why?

A rigid, restrictive, or bland diet was thought to be non-irritating to an ulcer and has been prescribed for decades. Experiments showed this approach didn't work. The result was an unhealed ulcer and an unhappy patient. A more liberal diet is used today. The patient is encouraged to eat any food he or she likes with a few exceptions—alcohol, coffee, meat extract (bouillon, gravy, broth), and black pepper.

Gone are the days of drinking heavy cream to "soothe" the ulcer, eating pureed fruits and vegetables, and avoiding gassy foods. Milk is not a good buffer and may stimulate acid secretion instead of decreasing it. A moderate amount of fiber is not irritating and helps avoid constipation. Each person reacts individually to gassy foods; what causes discomfort for one will not for another. Even eating frequent small meals has been challenged. Today there is no clear-cut diet treatment. The ulcer sufferer is encouraged to eat normally and simply avoid any food that causes him pain or discomfort. (See the following box "Have an Ulcer?" for some additional tips.)

FOOD ALLERGIES

* Are people intolerant to certain foods, and will these foods make them sick?

Actually there are three types of food intolerance that may occur:

Psychological food intolerance. Our cultural and reli-

HAVE AN ULCER?

<u>Do</u>	<u>Don't</u>
eat all foods you enjoy.	drink coffee, both regular and decaffeinated.
eat three meals a day.	drink alcohol.
eat calmly and slowly.	smoke.
	use aspirin.
	overeat.
	use meat extracts.
	use black pepper.
	eat before bedtime.

---

gious backgrounds form our food choices. A vegetarian forced to eat meat or an Orthodox Jew forced to eat pork might develop nausea and vomiting. You would probably gag at the thought of roast worms for dinner! Others avoid food because they fear it is unclean or may cause a disease such as cancer. These are all psychological rejections that you were *taught*. If you could put aside what you had learned, the vegetarian could eat meat, the Orthodox Jew could digest pork, and roast worms would be delectable. We hardly ever cast aside our values and beliefs and most of us avoid certain foods and never eat them. If questioned about the avoidance, some might say they are "intolerant" or "allergic." Rather than intolerance, a better description of this food avoidance might be a *food idiosyncrasy*—the refusal to eat a wholesome food. We all have a few idiosyncrasies.

Genetic food intolerance. Lactose intolerance, discomfort from drinking milk, is the classic example of a genetic food reaction. Sufferers cannot digest lactose (milk sugar) and have diarrhea, gas, cramping, and digestive upset. MSG intolerance is another. Often called "Chinese retaurant syndrome," sensitive people react to glutamate from the food additive monosodium glutamate (MSG). Both of these intolerances are discussed in more detail in Chapter 6.

Food allergy. After eating a particular food a person's

body may produce antibodies to that food, resulting in symptoms—wheezing, sneezing, diarrhea, hives, stomachaches, and in rare cases even shock and loss of consciousness. Why one person reacts to a food while others can eat it, is not known. The tendency toward allergies appears to be a family trait. Statistically, if allergy is present on one side of the family, a person has a 50 percent chance of being allergic to something at some point in his life. Allergy on both sides raises the risk to 75 percent. Many allergies occur in infants or in teens during puberty, but the hormonal changes of middle life can cause allergy symptoms for the first time. (See the following question for more information.)

* What is a food allergy?

Lots of people have food allergies, as many as 30 million. The reaction may be immediate (obvious), occurring a short time after eating. The shrimp-allergic person experiences hives, wheezing, headache, and other symptoms minutes after eating. More often the reaction is delayed (occult), which is less dramatic, more chronic, and harder to pinpoint. It occurs hours or even days later. A backache or joint pain may in fact be an allergic symptom that can be traced to a food eaten three to five days before.

A food allergy is seldom life threatening but it can be "life spoiling." Allergic people suffer a wide range of problems: digestive pain, nausea, heartburn, gas, diarrhea, constipation, nasal congestion, asthma, hives, skin inflammation, itching and scaling, headaches, muscle and joint aches, and bedwetting. Irrational and bizarre behavior resulting from a food allergy has tagged some as "neurotic." Since symptoms are so extensive and often happen long after eating the food, it is not surprising doctors dismiss the complaints and give them little attention. Attempts to desensitize a person to a food allergy are generally unsuccessful.

The chart "Food Allergies: The Common Offenders" will point out the more frequent food allergens and the symptoms they cause.

FOOD ALLERGIES: THE COMMON OFFENDERS

Food groups	*Some or all of these are possible reactions**

Milk
  whole
  dried
  skim
  buttermilk
  cheese
  custard
  cream
  creamed foods
  yogurt
  ice cream
  sherbet
  ice milk
  goat's milk
	Indigestion, constipation, diarrhea, gas, abdominal pain, nasal congestion, bronchial congestion, sore throat, ear inflammation, asthma, headache, bad breath, sweating, tension, fatigue.

Kola nut
  chocolate
  cola beverage (i.e., Coca-Cola, Pepsi, Tab)
	Headache, asthma, indigestion, chronic nasal inflammation, skin inflammation, itching.

Corn
  corn
  corn syrup
  corn cereal
  popcorn
  Cracker Jacks
  grits
  corn chips
  cornstarch
  cornmeal
  beer
  Canadian Whiskey
  bourbon whiskey
  corn oil[2]
	Irritability, insomnia, oversensitivity, restlessness, allergic fatigue,[1] headache, irritability, insomnia, restlessness.

* Note: Combinations of symptoms possible.
[1] Characterized by unresponsiveness, sleepiness, vague aching, weakness.
[2] Only an occasional offender.

Egg	Hives, eczema, asthma, indigestion, headache.
egg	
French toast	
baked goods	
icing	
meringue	
candies	
creamy salad dressing	
breaded food	
noodles	
egg substitutes	
vaccines grow in egg	
culture	
egg odor	

Pea family (legumes)[3]	Asthma, hives, headache.
peanut	
peanut butter	
dried peas	
dried beans	
honey[4]	
licorice	
soybean	
soy flour	
soy protein	
soy milk	
soy oil[1]	
alfalfa	

Citrus fruits[5]	Eczema, hives, asthma, canker sores.
orange	
lemon	
lime	
grapefruit	
tangerine	

[3] Reactions to this group are severe, including shock.

[4] In the U.S., honey is gathered primarily from plants in this family (i.e., clover, alfalfa).

[5] If the person is sensitive to citric acid he or she will also react to tart artificial drinks and pineapple.

Food groups	Some or all of these are possible reactions*

Tomato
  ketchup
  chili
  prepared foods
	Eczema, hives, asthma, mouth soreness.

Wheat and small grains[3]
  rice
  barley
  oats
  wild rice
  millet
  rye[2]
	Asthma, indigestion, eczema, nasal congestion, bronchial congestion.

Cinnamon[6]
  ketchup
  chewing gum
  candies
  baked goods
  applesauce
  apple pies and cakes
  chili
  luncheon meats
  pumpkin pies and cakes
	Hives, headache, asthma.

Artificial food colors
  red dye amaranth
  yellow dye tartrazine
    colored foods
    colored drinks
    colored medicines
	Asthma, hives

[6] Cinnamon-sensitive patients cannot tolerate bay leaf.

PSORIASIS

* Can I treat my psoriasis with a diet change?

Even though many diet remedies have been tried, none have given the psoriasis sufferer lasting results. The condition causes skim inflammation and scaling. At times psoriasis causes discomfort while at other times it seems to improve. Low-protein diets and diets high in turkey have provided some with relief, as have diets low in fruits, nuts, corn, milk, coffee, soda, tomatoes, and pineapple.

All these diets were tried on only a few people and the success is difficult to evaluate since the condition is complicated and may have spontaneous improvement unrelated to treatment. Avoiding a large group of foods, hoping for relief, may lead to poor diet and poor health. A low animal protein diet with generous use of vegetable proteins may give some relief and will cause no nutrient imbalances. A psoriasis sufferer might try this approach.

DIVERTICULITIS

* What is diverticulitis?

Diverticulosis is a condition in which the walls of the large intestine form blowouts or outpouching in weakened spots. The pouches are called *diverticula*. They may become inflamed or infected. If that happens, the condition is called *diverticulitis*. It's painful and may also cause nausea, vomiting, gas, and fever. Diverticulitis is dangerous since the weak spots or outpouches in the intestine could rupture. Only 10 to 15 percent of those with diverticulosis suffer diverticulitis.

Diet has been used successfully to prevent, treat, and eliminate this problem, which occurs more frequently as we get older. (See the following question for more information.)

* Should I eat only pureed, bland foods if I have diverticulitis?

Traditionally this was the treatment and it is used today when a person has a full-blown painful episode. However, for prevention of discomfort and to prevent further damage to the intestine, a moderate-to high-fiber diet is recommended. Some feel diverticulosis results from chronic constipation and straining. Those who eat a large proportion of refined foods and little fiber seem to suffer the most.

A diet with ample fiber (fruits, vegetables, whole-grain breads, and cereals) will prevent constipation by helping to move the stool through the bowel quickly. This puts less strain on the intestinal wall and reduces the chance of residue being caught in the outpouches (diverticula), cutting down on the risk of infection. Bran is especially useful in producing a large, soft stool that can be easily passed. For more information, see the highlight box "Bothered by Diverticulosis?" (Look over Chapter 6 for hints on adding fiber to the diet and eliminating constipation. See also Chapter 1's section on Fiber.)

BOTHERED BY DIVERTICULOSIS?

_Do_
eat foods high in fiber
   (whole-grain breads and
   cereals, fruits, vegetables).
add one to two teaspoons of
   bran to each meal.
drink six to eight glasses of
   liquid a day.
eat bland, refined foods
   during painful periods.

Don't
strain at the stool.

use laxatives.

GALLBLADDER DISEASE

* How do you get gallstones?

It's been estimated that 12 million women and 4 million men in the United States have gallstones. Over half don't even know it because they have no symptoms. Gallstones form when the gallbladder does not work properly. This can occur as we age or it can be due to an infection of the gallbladder. Continually eating high-fat foods, being overweight, taking estrogens, having many children, or having low levels of HDL cholesterol, can increase the likelihood of forming gallstones.

When gallstones are present the condition is called "cholelithiasis" and may require surgery to remove the gallbladder. In other instances the stones may be dissolved with drugs. Gallstones are almost pure cholesterol since cholesterol is used to manufacture bile, which is stored in the gallbladder. When functioning normally the gallbladder concentrates bile and delivers it to the small intestine, as needed, to digest fat. When inflammed, the gallbladder does not work properly and cholesterol settles out of the bile solution, forming gallstones. If the stones block the passageway to the intestines, pain results. Often there is a feeling of extreme fullness and bloating after eating. Many will have difficulty digesting fatty foods. (See the following question for more information.)

* My doctor wants to remove my gallbladder. How will I digest food afterward?

The gallbladder does not digest food. It is a concentrating and holding tank for bile. Bile, which breaks up fat and prepares it for easy digestion, is made in the liver. After gallbladder surgery, the bile is stored in a duct between the liver and the intestine. This duct stretches to increase its holding capacity. Immediately after surgery and for a few months thereafter, you need to eat a diet low in fat. (See the question "The doctor put my husband on a low-fat diet. . . ." in Chapter 8's Fat section for information on what foods to eat.) As the surgery heals and the bile duct stretches, fat digestion returns to normal. For good health it is wise never to return to a high-fat diet, but in three or four months you should be eating everything without pain or indigestion.

DIABETES

* What is diabetes?

Diabetes, or more correctly, diabetes mellitus, refers to a condition where there are high levels of sugar (glucose) in the blood. Some of that sugar is passed out in the urine and this is the reason for the name. *Diabetes mellitus* means "passing honey" in a mixture of Greek and Latin. This is also the reason that excessive thirst may be a symptom of diabetes.

Insulin, a hormone made by the pancreas, is needed for the body to use glucose normally. The reason for the high glucose level in the blood is either that little or no insulin is produced or that the insulin produced is inactive. In other words, the diabetic cannot use glucose normally; this is referred to as *glucose intolerance.*

There are two general types of diabetes. People who have Type I need to take insulin, to control the condition, while others, with the more common kind, Type II, often can be helped by weight loss (if needed) and eating a nutritionally adequate, balanced diet low in sweets. Most people who become diabetic after age forty have Type II.

The incidence of diabetes increases as people age. In the twenty-five-to-forty-four-year-old age group, seventeen out of one thousand are diabetic while at age sixty-five to seventy-four, there are seventy-nine per thousand. (See the following question for more information.)

* My mother is a diabetic. Does that mean I will become one too?

Most researchers agree that at least the predisposition to diabetes is inherited. But whether or not a predisposed person develops the disease depends on many factors. Excess food, obesity, acute stress, and changes in other hormones in the body can "unmask" the diabetes.

There is greater risk for developing diabetes if you are overweight. In fact, the risk doubles for every 20 percent of excess weight. Because you have a family history of diabetes, it is wise for you to have regular checkups and keep your weight normal. You can do that by avoiding excess calories and exercising regularly.

* What should diabetics eat?

They should eat the same moderate-calorie diet anyone else eats. It should be relatively high in complex carbohydrate (starch), low in fat (saturated fat in particular), and moderately high in protein. A good distribution is 30 percent fat,

15 to 20 percent protein, and 50 to 55 percent carbohydrate. As an example, a 1,600 Calorie diet divided up like this would have 60 grams of protein, 220 grams of carbohydrate, and 55 grams of fat. These diets are easily followed when the allowed foods are given in exchanges. (See Appendix C.)

Diabetics should avoid all sugar and foods that are made with it. Fiber has been shown to improve the diabetic's ability to handle sugar. High-fiber foods should be included. Depending on the diabetic's condition and the drug used (if any), alcohol can be used in moderation. It can be substituted for some of the day's calories, as long as the calorie allowance is more than 1,500. If it is less than that, it will be difficult to use some of the calories for alcohol and still have enough left to provide all necessary nutrients. (See the question "As a diabetic, can't I have an occasional glass of wine or beer?" in Chapter 4.)

* My husband is a recently diagnosed diabetic. Why was he given a diet high in carbohydrates?

You may have always heard that diabetics should not eat carbohydrates. We know now that this restriction is not necessary. In fact, when you increase the amount of carbohydrate a diabetic eats, you actually improve his or her glucose tolerance or ability to use carbohydrate. Instead of limiting carbohydrate it is more important to limit total calories and fat.

You must remember, though, that the carbohydrates your husband should eat are starches, not refined sugars. Sweets like candy, pastries, doughnuts, and pudding should not be a part of your husband's diet. The sugars in fruits, in moderation, are all right because they come packaged with fiber and nutrients needed for health.

* Now that I'm a diabetic can I still enjoy an occasional fast food meal?

Yes, you can. Many diabetics eat one meal a day in fast food restaurants. Appendix D lists the Fast Food Exchanges for Diabetics and Dieters. This will help you to choose foods so that you can stay within your allotted exchanges for the day.

When you have enjoyed a fast food meal be sure that fruit, vegetables, and milk are included in other meals so that you will be getting all the nutrients you need for good health.

✻ I heard on the radio that a chromium supplement can cure my diabetes. How much should I take?

Chromium, protein, and niacin make up the glucose tolerance factor (GTF). This factor helps the body use glucose normally by increasing the activity of insulin. Some diabetics who were deficient in chromium improved their ability to use glucose after they were given chromium supplements. That does not mean that they were cured, only that their condition was made less severe. If you have normal levels of chromium in your body, additional supplements *will not* improve your diabetes.

Good sources of chromium are eggs, liver, potatoes (with skin), nuts, black pepper, and whole grains. You would need to eat four slices of white bread to get the chromium in one slice of whole wheat. Brewer's yeast also is a source of chromium. Don't waste your money buying the glucose tolerance factor supplement sold in health food stores, as this is derived from yeast and is useful only to yeast, not to you.

✻ If I am a diabetic can I eat "dietetic candy" and chew "sugarless" gum?

Dietetic candy and sugarless gum are usually sweetened with saccharin and sorbitol or mannitol. Xylitol is only found in gums and breath mints. Sorbitol, mannitol, and xylitol are sugar alcohols, a chemical form of sugar with the same calorie content as table sugar (sucrose). Xylitol is as sweet as table sugar but sorbitol and mannitol are only half as sweet, and that is why they are almost always coupled with saccharin in dietetic "sweets."

A well-controlled diabetic can use these substitute sweeteners because they are absorbed slowly and used in the body almost completely without the need for insulin. However, the picture is not as rosy as it may seem. The diabetic cannot use these sugar substitutes freely. They contribute calories, the same as regular sugar. They are less sweet than sugar, so more is needed to achieve the same degree of sweetness. The safety of xylitol is currently an unclear issue. Its use will remain limited until conclusive results on its safety are proven. And most importantly, these sugar alcohols can all cause stomach cramps and diarrhea. "Chewing gum diarrhea" or "dietetic food diarrhea," as the condition is known, is so prevalent among chronic users that food labels must carry a warning about this possible effect. A dose of 20 or more grams a day (about four teaspoons) can cause problems. You could get this much sorbitol if you ate one roll of dietetic mints and one dietetic candy bar. (For more information see next question. Also see "When I'm trying to lose weight is fructose better for me . . ." in Chapter 7 in the section on Diet, Exercise, and Pills.)

* If I buy "dietetic" foods will they help me to control my diabetes?

The FDA (Food and Drug Administration) recently set up new labeling rules that restrict the use of the terms "diet," "dietetic," and "sugarless." Foods packaged for use by diabetics, such as gelatin desserts, cakes, candy, cookies, ice cream, and syrups, must have the following label statement: DIABETICS: THIS PRODUCT MAY BE USEFUL IN YOUR DIET ON THE ADVICE OF YOUR PHYSICIAN. When this statement does not appear, the food may be low in calories but contain sugar and would not be suitable for your use.

There is nothing wrong with dietetic foods and sometimes they replace regular items you may no longer use. Remember, however, that they are not necessary and you can plan suitable and tasty meals without them.

Diet sodas are not regulated under these new rules. However, their labeling requirements have been such that they have always listed the percentage of saccharin and presence of sorbitol, mannitol, sugar, or carbohydrates. You can easily determine what is in a particular brand simply by reading the label. (See the chart "Saccharine in Soda and Sweeteners" in Chapter 7 and the questions in that chapter on pages 194 and 196.)

HYPOGLYCEMIA

* My neighbor says she has hypoglycemia. What is this?

Hypoglycemia occurs when a person has a lower than normal level of blood sugar (glucose). Because the symptoms—sweating, shaking, dizziness, hunger, tiredness—are so common, many people mistakenly believe they have hypoglycemia. There are a very few people who regularly produce too much insulin so that their blood sugar is abnormally low. Such a condition can be diagnosed by repeated glucose tolerance tests. Eating high-protein foods, fewer carbohydrates, and avoiding sugar completely can relieve the symptoms.

Temporary cases of hypoglycemia are more usual. These can be caused by skipping a meal, eating large amounts of carbohydrate foods, or substituting alcoholic drinks for a meal. (Anxiety can produce similar symptoms.) These occasional instances can be handled by eating a balanced meal or snack, not a sweet.

CANCER

* What is cancer?

Cancer is not a simple disease. There are *cancers* which include various tumors and neoplasms (new growth) that grow in different sites in the body in an uncontrolled manner. When a cancer grows it interferes with the normal functioning of an organ or tissue and its growth is difficult to stop. A cancer cell is derived from a normal cell that has lost control over cell reproduction. The normal cell develops into a cancer cell because of an initiating event. Several factors can cause this loss of normal cell control.

Radiation may alter cell reproduction, either general atmospheric radiation that is always present, or exposure to industrial or medical radiation. Or the cancer may be initiated by a *carcinogen* that enters the cell and alters it. (See the following question.)

After the initiating event, many things may happen. Healthy cells have an automatic immune response to foreign substances and may destroy the cancer before it can grow. At times the immunological system appears not to work against the cancer, leading some researchers to speculate that cancer may be a failure of our immune system. If the cancer is not destroyed it will grow, in some, slowly, taking many years to make itself known. In others the growth is rapid.

✻ What is a carcinogen?

A carcinogen is a cancer-causing substance. Results from animal studies and other research have shown about thirty substances cause cancer, or are suspected of causing cancer, in people. Carcinogens may be man-made or naturally occurring chemicals in food, air, water, or the workplace.

Food often acts as a carrier, transporting a carcinogen into the body. The carcinogen may be a nutrient, an additive, or an accidental contaminant such as pesticide residue. Benzopyrene, nitrites, cyclamates, sassafras, and DES (diethylstilbestrol) have all been suspected of carcinogenicity. When the link between cancer and a chemical appears strong, the chemical will be labeled a carcinogen and removed from our food supply as mandated by the Delaney Clause of the Federal Food, Drug, and Cosmetics Act.

It must be stressed that not all chemicals are carcinogenic. In fact, relatively few are. Most chemicals, even those that are toxic and dangerous, do not cause cancer. (See Appendix B, "Natural Toxins in Food," for information on naturally occurring carcinogens.)

✻ Can a poor diet cause cancer?

Studies of cancer trends in populations suggest that diet affects more than half of all cancers in women and at least one-third of all cancers in men. Some feel the diet-cancer relationship may be even greater than this. There appears to be three ways that nutrition may initiate cancer. First, the food may carry the carcinogen into the body. Second, nutrient deficiency may favor cancer development. Third, excess nutrients—protein, fat, vitamins, or minerals—may alter body functioning and induce cancer growth.

Colon cancer rates increase with low-fiber diets or high-meat intakes. Breast cancer rates correlate with high-fat intake and low-fiber diets. Abuse of alcohol seems to promote cancers of the digestive tract, although alcohol itself is not carcinogenic. Deficiencies of trace minerals, like selenium, have been linked to an increased risk of cancer. Chronic vitamin deficiencies result in more tumor growth in animals.

Other studies reveal some positive facts about nutrition and cancer that are worth noting. In the United States there has been a sharp decrease in stomach cancer although pollution has increased. It appears that our safe and clean food supply is the protective factor. A number of natural and artificial antioxidants—vitamins E and C, selenium, BHT, and BHA (see question "Do food additives cause cancer?")—protect against carcinogens in a way yet to be determined. Certain plants and naturally occurring substances in food may be able to inhibit cancer cells. Brussels sprouts, cabbage, cauliflower, broccoli, carotene, and chlorophyll have been successful in animal experiments. Of all diet modifications that have been tried, the one that has had the most constant effect on inhibiting cancer growth is a low-calorie intake.

Based on all we currently know about cancer and nutrition, the best advice we can give is to eat a wide variety of food in a low-calorie diet.

* Can a change in what I eat reduce my risk of stomach cancer?

We have a low rate of stomach cancer in the United States but some authorities feel it could be even lower if we changed our diet in five ways.

1. Reduce nitrate exposure. We get nitrates in cured meat (such as ham and bacon), in some vegetables (spinach, carrots, beets, radishes, celery, and lettuce), and in drinking water. Approximately 5 percent of the communities in the United States have high nitrate levels in their water supply.

2. Lower salt intake. Some research has suggested that high levels of sodium (salt is sodium chloride) promote cancer formation.

3. Increase intake of vitamin C.

4. Raise the protein to starch ratio in the diet. Consuming a low-protein diet is not typical in the U.S., so this point poses little risk.

5. Encourage good dental hygiene. Bacteria, commonly found in the mouth, are able to convert nitrate to nitrite, which is then swallowed in the saliva.

* I am undergoing treatment for cancer and find eating is unpleasant. What can you suggest?

Although we have made advances in the treatment of some forms of cancer, the treatment itself causes side effects that make eating unpleasant. Foods you enjoyed may taste strange and you suffer priods of nausea, vomiting, and a sore mouth.

The bitter taste sensation may be magnified, causing meat to have an aftertaste. Poultry, fish, eggs, and cheese are more appealing. Very cold meats or meats with a sweet sauce (plum or peach) are more acceptable. You might find you like things sweeter than normal. If so, sweeten to taste. Sprinkle extra sugar on your cereal or dessert and even try some experimenting, like a little brown sugar in mashed potatoes. Salty and sour tastes usually remain normal. Use these flavors to enhance your meals. Try seasoning with soy sauce. For snacks you may enjoy a pickled salad, pretzels, or salted nuts.

Smells may be troublesome too. If possible, stay out of the kitchen during cooking or cook with a window open and a kitchen fan on. Try eating in another room.

The most important thing to keep in mind is that eating is part of your treatment, which will be more successful if you are well nourished. Try any tricks that work for you no matter how absurd. The following chart "Dealing with the Discomforts of Cancer Treatment" might provide some clues.

Dealing with the Discomfort of Cancer Treatment

Discomfort	Food suggestions
Thick, sticky saliva	Use liquid foods (soups, drinks, pureed fruits). Use hot tea with lemon or suck on sour lemon drops. Eat a light breakfast.
Dry mouth (xerostomia)	Serve foods with sauces, broth, or gravies. Serve plenty of liquids along with meals. Practice good dental care. Increase saliva flow by using sugarless lemon drops or gum, lemon tea, lemonade, sports gum (Gatorade Gum), or artificial saliva substitute.
Diarrhea	Drink ample liquids such as water, fruit ades, and low-acid fruit juices (apricot, peach, pear). Eat food low in fiber. Use soybean milk if regular milk causes discomfort. Eat foods high in potassium.*
Nausea and vomiting	Do not eat for several hours before treatment. Salty or cold foods control nausea and vomiting. Do not eat sweet or greasy foods. Do not mix hot and cold foods. Do not drink rapidly. Eat slowly. Eat small meals. Lie down or rest after eating.

Mouth blindness (dysgeusia)	Use odor, texture, and eye appeal to encourage eating. Select strongly flavored foods (barbecue and steak sauce). Acid foods, like lemonade, stimulate taste.
Sore mouth and esophagus	Eat soft, bland food; avoid rough, raw, and spicy foods. Rinse several times a day with a solution of salt, water, and sodium bicarbonate.
Constipation	Eat high-fiber food if chewing and swallowing are not a problem. Use bran added to cooked food. Drink prune juice. Drink 8 or more glasses liquid each day. Have regular, daily exercise.

* See page 109 for a list of foods high in potassium.

* Do food additives cause cancer?

One out of two people believe food additives are a major cause of cancer. Yet a recent analysis of cancer trends states that food additives are responsible for less than 1 percent of all cancer and that some additives may in fact provide cancer protection.

BHA (butylated hydroxyanisole) and BHT (butylated hydroxytoluene) are antioxidants added to processed foods to prevent fats from becoming rancid. Both have been under fire and there was great pressure to remove them from our food supply. Research, however, has revealed that both BHA and BHT may protect against tumor formation in some unknown way.

In spite of this, additives should be carefully scrutinized for safety. The FDA regulates the approval of any new additives proposed. This regulation is so strict that polydextrose, a bulking agent that was approved in 1981, was the first major food additive introduced into our food supply in five years. Additives currently in use and considered GRAS (Generally Recognized As Safe) have just undergone an extensive re-evaluation. Of the 415 additives on the GRAS list, only 305 were considered safe. The remaining ones were classified so that additional research or regulation could be imposed upon them. Many of these, such as saccharin and caffeine, are now being regulated under an interim status requiring more study. A small group will require even tighter regulation or removal from the food supply. The FDA will implement all these findings over the next two years.

Food colors as a group have been hardest hit by the new tighter regulation. Currently, only seven colors are permitted in the U.S. food supply: Red No. 3, Blue No. 2, Yellow No. 5, Green No. 3, Yellow No. 6, Blue No. 1, and Red No. 40. Red No. 2, removed in 1976, recently showed some anticancer properties in animal studies.

There is still much we need to learn about additives, their interaction in the body, and their effect on cancer. Although the risk is small, to protect yourself against possible harm from food additives eat a wide variety of food so that no one substance will be eaten in large enough amounts to create a hazard to your health. (See Appendix E for additional information on food additives.)

* Is it true that tea with lemon causes cancer?

A laboratory experiment showed that when tea with lemon added was drunk from a Styrofoam (polystyrene) cup, a large amount of the container was dissolved into the tea. Tea with lemon erodes the Styrofoam container and may chemically combine with it. Since polystyrene is a known carcinogen for laboratory animals, we suggest reviving the tradition of drinking tea with lemon from fine china cups.

* Do broiled hamburgers cause cancer?

Hamburgers have been under fire lately for their possible role in cancer promotion. Mutagens and benzopyrene, substances with carcinogenic (cancer-promoting) potential, have been isolated from the hamburger.

Mutagens, chemical compounds that cause inherited or genetic changes, are found only in *cooked* hamburgers. Most known mutagens are carcinogenic to laboratory animals. The mutagens form when the hamburgers are cooked in a frying pan, on a griddle or in an electric hamburger cooker at high temperatures. It is thought that the beef undergoes a chemical reaction resulting in mutagens, since raw hamburger does not contain any. When a hamburger is cooked under an electric broiler or a microwave oven (without using the ceramic "browning tray") no mutagens form. Deep-fat frying will not promote mutagen formation. In hamburgers mutagens are potentially carcinogenic to people, but whether the risk is great, small, or nonexistent is yet to be determined.

Since 1933, it's been known that benzopyrene will cause cancer in lab animals. In 1963, benzopyrene was found in broiled meat. Hamburgers, T-bone steak, fish, pork chops, and chicken have all had measurable levels after broiling. What appears to increase the benzopyrene levels in these meats is the type of broiling. Charcoal broiling causes the greatest formation and is the single largest source of benzopyrene in food. It is formed when charcoal burns and the smoke deposits on the meat, when fat drips on the coals and vaporizes, or when the flames touch the meat. Placing a pan or aluminum foil between the meat and the charcoal smoke and flames substantially reduces benzopyrene levels. Cooking in a broiler with the heat source *above* the meat eliminates the formation of the carcinogen. Once again, the method of cooking can be changed to reduce the risk.

* Can Laetrile cure cancer?

Laetrile is derived from the apricot pit and is the most widely pushed unproven anticancer drug. The substance

has received publicity and has been backed by many promi-
nent people. The theory behind it suggests that there is only
one kind of cancer and this miracle drug can destroy those
cells.

An extensive study on the effectiveness of Laetrile in cancer treatment has been completed and reported in the *New
England Journal of Medicine*. It showed no benefit in cures,
improvements, or stabilization of cancer. What it did show is
that Laetrile is toxic and patients who elect to use it run the
risk of cyanide poisoning.

Laetrile's main constituent, *amygdalin*, is a chemical
found in peach, apricot, apple, plum, and bitter almond pits.
Amygdalin is a cyanide compound and causes poisoning and
death if taken in large amounts. The FDA banned foods containing amygdalin and supplements marketed as B_{17}. Tablets, liquid, and granular Laetrile can cause acute or chronic
poisoning. Injected Laetrile is less toxic. The decision to use
Laetrile treatment belongs to the patient, who should know
that research does not support its curative properties and that
he or she runs the risk of cyanide poisoning.

* Can vitamin B_{15} prevent cancer?

No, because there is no such vitamin as B_{15}. The substance marketed as B_{15} is calcium pangamate or pangamic
acid, chemical substances that have no vitaminlike activity in
the body. The terms "B_{15}" and "pangamate" were coined in
the early 1950s by the scientist E. T. Krebs to name a substance he had isolated from apricot pits and used for the
treatment of cancer.

Supporters claim B_{15} increases oxygen uptake by blood
and tissues, which results in more energy and lowered blood
cholesterol among other benefits. It is being promoted as a
cure for heart disease, diabetes, glaucoma, alcoholism, liver
disease, allergies, and arthritis. None of these claims are sup-
ported by research. Some B_{15} ads even claim that it "slows
down the aging process." One B_{15} manufacturer uses a quote
from a Russian scientist who allegedly said "the day will
come when pangamic acid will be next to the saltshaker in

every home with people over forty." At \$8 or more per one hundred tablets, B_{15} promoters surely hope this will be the case.

B_{15} cannot be considered harmless. Laboratory tests show it may cause mutations. In large doses one B_{15} chemical (diisoproplyammonium dichloroacetate) can be harmful to those with low blood pressure or circulatory problems.

The B_{15} saga is a classic example of a consumer health fraud. Don't fall for it.

* Are coffee enemas useful in treating cancer?

Coffee enemas are recommended for cancer, diverticulitis, and other chronic conditions. Their value as a treatment is questionable since extensive use has caused death in a few cases.

These enemas, more correctly called "colonic irrigations," are supposed to remove toxic substances from the body. To do this, huge amounts of fluid are slowly pushed into the large intestines. The enemas may be given as frequently as every two hours. One famous case centered around a well-known actor, now deceased, who sought this treatment for chest cancer.

Naturopathic physicians may specialize in colonics, charging up to \$30 for a whopping enema. Beside being costly, the treatment is unsafe, causing damage to the bowel and imbalances in the body's minerals and fluid, which may result in death. Colonic irrigation, made of coffee or of any other solution, must be considered an unproven method for cancer care and life threatening as well.

10

A Simple Guide to Vegetarian Eating

Many of you may think of vegetarians as the flower children of the 1960s. Although the spirit of the 60s and 70s reawakened interest in vegetarian eating, vegetarianism is not a fad. The popularity of vegetarianism is greater today than it has been at any time in our nation's history. Even those who are not total vegetarians have felt the impact of this way of eating—less red meat, more whole grains, more fresh foods, and less fat.

Vegetarianism—the abstinence from flesh foods—is as old as mankind. Prehistoric man was basically vegetarian, searching out plants, seeds, and roots. Meat was an occasional luxury. Many argue that the original diet set forth in the Bible was meatless and only after the deluge, when vegetation was destroyed, did man begin eating meat. The Buddhists, Egyptians, Greeks, Romans, and early Christians all had noted leaders who favored abstinence from meat. The idea of vegetarianism survived through time in many religious groups—Hindus, Buddhist monks, Trappist monks, and Yemenite Jews—all of whose roots lie in ancient teachings.

During the Renaissance, Bacon, Shakespeare, Milton, Voltaire, and others, though not all vegetarians, fought against the slaughter of animals and favored a "return to nature." Even Benjamin Franklin advocated a diet that was simpler and less rich.

274

The 1800s witnessed a resurgence in vegetarianism much like today. Reuben Mussey, the fourth president of the American Medical Association and Edward Hitchcock, president of Amherst College, were advocates, as were Sylvester Graham, of graham cracker fame, and Dr. Harvey Kellogg, of cereal fame. Dr. Kellogg established the Battle Creek Sanitarium in Michigan to cure disease with a meatless diet. This period also saw the beginning of the Seventh-Day Adventists Church, which preaches voluntary exclusion of meat and meat products. The church flourishes today, with third- and fourth-generation vegetarians and an elaborate network of educational systems and qualified medical professionals to assist members. Loma Linda University, an arm of the church, has a School of Public Health that has contributed outstanding research on the health of vegetarians.

Seventh-Day Adventists are quite healthy—leaner than their meat-eating counterparts, with lowered cholesterol values, less incidence of heart disease, breast and lung cancer, diabetes, and osteoporosis. Their superior health is attributed to the limited use of alcohol, tobacco, and animal products. They are surely a testimonial to the value of vegetarianism.

Knowing this, should we all give up meat forever? After you read this chapter, we won't take a head count of converts but we do hope it will spark your imagination and entice you to experiment with an occasional nonmeat meal. We have enlarged our menu planning to regularly include many foods once considered "vegetarian."

* Exactly what is a vegetarian?

By definition a *vegetarian* is "one who lives wholly or principally on vegetable foods; a person who, on principle, abstains from any form of animal food. . . ." The reasons for not eating meat are almost as numerous as the people who practice it—religion, culture, "respect for life," ecological or environmental principles, self-discipline, economics, health, a method of protest, or a quest for longevity.

Todays "vegetarians" share no common food habits or philosophical bonds. They can come from any socioeconomic level and include old and young alike, cutting across all cultural groups. Their only common bond is their choice of a vegetarian diet. Some have been life-long vegetarians but most are new adherents or partial vegetarians, excluding some groups of animal food but not all. Today's vegetarian approaches his or her diet in a very individual fashion. One may simply exclude red meats, finding poultry and fish acceptable. Another may eat eggs, cheese, and milk but refuse all meat products. A few are total vegetarians, eating only plant foods. The total practice takes thought and planning but it can lead to a healthy diet. We'll address that more fully in another question. A small group eats selections of foods that are limited and may be bizarre. These patterns can have serious consequences and have led to deficiency diseases and even death. (See the question "What are macrobiotic foods?" in this chapter.)

Let's take a closer look at the different types of vegetarian diets.

Vegan or total vegetarian—a person who eats only plant food.

Lactovegetarian—a person who eats plant food, milk, and milk products (cheese, yogurt, ice cream, pudding, etc.).

Lacto-ovo-vegetarian—a person who eats plant food, milk and milk products, and eggs (meat, poultry, fish, and seafood are excluded; this is a nonflesh diet).

Semivegetarian or partial vegetarian—a person who eats some animal or fish foods but not all of them; this group includes "nonred meat eaters" who may or may not include one or all of the following in their diet: eggs, poultry, cheese, milk, fish, and seafood.

✳ What do vegetarians eat?

Food, much like you and I, except they rely on grains, eggs and dairy products to provide protein. Meat eaters rely on these also but get most of their protein from meat, poultry, and fish. The basic four food groups—milk, meat, fruits and vegetables, and grains—are the same for everyone. The vegetarian makes some adjustments in the meat group and increases the number of servings from the other groups. (See the chart "Vegetarian Four Food Groups.")

VEGETARIAN FOUR FOOD GROUPS

Milk (Use low-fat or 2% milk and milk products)
2 or more servings daily
1 serving = 1 cup milk
1 cup milk = 1½ ounces cheese
          = 2 cups cottage cheese
          = 1 cup pudding
          = 1 cup custard
          = 1 cup yogurt
          = 1½ cups ice cream
          = 1 cup cooked collard greens
          = 1½ cups cooked kale, mustard greens, dandelion greens
          = 2 cups okra
          = 1⅓ cups cooked bok choy
          = 2½ ounces sardines

Legumes*, Nuts, Seeds, and Eggs (Meat Substitutes)
2 servings daily
1 serving = 1 cup legumes
          = ¼ cup peanut butter
          = 6 ounces tofu (soybean curd)
          = 2 eggs
          = 2 slices cheese
          = ½ cup cottage cheese
          = 1½ ounce or 3 tablespoons nuts or seeds

* Dried peas, beans and peanuts.

Fruits and Vegetables

4 or more servings daily. A food rich in vitamin C is recommended daily

1 serving = 1 medium whole fruit or vegetable (raw or cooked)
        = ½ cup cooked vegetable or fruit
        = ½ large fruit (i.e., grapefruit)
        = 2 to 3 small fruits (i.e., plum)
        = ½ cup (4 ounces) juice
        = 2 tablespoons dried fruit
        = 1 cup raw bulky or leaf vegetable (i.e., spinach or bean sprouts)

Grains—Bread, Cereal, Pasta, Rice

6 or more servings daily

1 serving = 1 slice of bread
        = 1 cup cold cereal
        = ½ cup cooked cereal
        = ¼ to ⅓ cup granola-type cereal
        = 1 tablespoon wheat germ
        = ¾ cup brown rice
        = ¾ cup pasta or noodles
        = 1 biscuit, muffin, or pancake
        = 1 slice nut or fruit bread
        = 4 crackers
        = 1 tablespoon nutritional yeast

* Are vegetarians healthy?

Becoming and remaining a vegetarian adds as much as ten years to your expected life-span by reducing your risk of obesity, diabetes, heart disease, cancer, and osteoporosis. We'd call that healthy!

Vegetarians are leaner than most meat eaters by an average of ten to twenty pounds. Even those who became vegetarians late in life report a weight loss rather than gain. Switching from a reliance on animal protein to a diet high in legumes, grains, and other plant foods will lower cholesterol and the risk of heart disease. Even lacto-ovo-vegetarians have significantly lower cholesterol values and risk rates. Strong scientific evidence linking vegetarianism and a lowered risk of cancer is still to be found. In the meantime, the small number of cancers among this group continually points to a link.

Osteoporosis, bone thinning, is a major health problem we face as we get older. For meat eaters trouble starts after forty and gets progressively worse. (See Chapter 5, Osteoporosis and Calcium section.) Vegetarians have 50 percent less bone loss at age sixty and have consistently thicker and stronger bones—up to the age of eighty-nine.

A well-planned vegetarian diet, especially one that includes milk and eggs, easily meets all our nutritional needs and may provide us with an even better state of health.

* Do vegetarians lack any vitamins because they do not eat meat?

A lacto-ovo-vegetarian diet easily meets all your needs and may provide some health benefits as well. A total vegetarian (a vegan) must plan more carefully, as all protein is from plant sources. Vitamin B_{12} and vitamin D may be in short supply since there is no good source of these in plant foods.

Nutritional yeast (grown on a B_{12}-enriched media), fortified soy milk, or a supplement are the easiest ways to get B_{12}. Cold breakfast cereals also provide some, about 25 percent of the RDA in one serving. The exceptions to this are Product 19, Total, and Most, providing 100 percent of the RDA for B_{12} in a serving. Seaweed and algae contaminated by plankton may have some B_{12} content but this source is variable and should not be relied on solely. A small amount of vitamin B_{12} is made in the body, and food contaminated with mold or insects is another source.

Vitamin D is found in fortified soy milk, in breakfast cereals, and in cod liver oil. It can be made in the body (the sunshine vitamin) when you spend enough time outdoors. The sun should not be relied on as the only source.

A higher fiber intake might block mineral absorption and some questions have been raised about iron, calcium, and zinc. However, it appears an adaptive mechanism is set in motion and mineral deficiency is not a concern to most healthy vegetarians.

As with the general population, bizarre eating habits or a narrow selection of food may cause problems. Eating a wide variety of foods in moderate amounts provides the vegetarian with all his or her nutritional needs.

* How can a vegetarian get enough protein if he or she doesn't eat meat?

Protein is found in many foods besides meat—poultry, fish, milk, and dairy foods, eggs, legumes, grains, nuts, and seeds. Even if no meat is eaten, vegetarians will eat some if not all of the other protein sources. Poultry, fish, dairy foods, and eggs are excellent quality proteins. If these are included in a meal, protein will be ample.

Legumes, grains, nuts, and seeds are good but not equal to meat or other animal proteins. To assure enough protein at each meal the vegetarian needs to couple at least two of these to supply the same protein found in one animal source. For example, if you eliminate the lamb chop from the following meal:

Lamb chop
Baked winter squash
Steamed broccoli
Tossed salad
Dinner roll

you'd need to replace it with *two* vegetable proteins to equal the protein value of the lamb chop:

Rice and lentils
Baked winter squash
Steamed broccoli
Tossed salad
Dinner roll

This use of two or more vegetable proteins in one meal is called *complementation*—the sum of the proteins eaten at the same time. You can achieve the same result with a small amount of animal protein coupled with a vegetable protein—cereal plus milk.

You complement protein all the time without trying to:

Macaroni and cheese = grain + dairy food
Peanut butter on whole-wheat bread = legume + grain
Buckwheat pancakes = grain + egg + milk
Rice au gratin = grain + dairy food
Yogurt and wheat germ = dairy + grain
Rice pudding = grain + dairy
Minestrone soup = grain + legumes
Walnut bread = nut + grain

There are six protein categories that a vegetarian may draw from—grains, legumes, dairy foods, eggs, nuts, and seeds. A simple rule is to eat at least two of these categories at each meal to be sure you are getting the correct amount and type of protein you need.

Two charts should interest you. "Protein in Foods," Chapter 1, shows what foods give us protein and how much each contributes to the diet. "Complement Your Proteins" in this section shows protein categories that may be combined to replace meat or to limit its use in meals. Serving chopped meat as a hamburger, you'd need 4 ounces of raw meat to cook a meal-size burger. Combine that same 4 ounces into chili with red kidney beans and you can serve four people. You complemented a small amount of meat protein with a generous amount of vegetable protein. Omit the meat and serve the chili over rice and you are still providing a good main dish protein source.

* I see breakfast "sausages" which are not made of meat. Should I buy them?

These "sausages" and other nonmeat "meats" currently found in the supermarket are plant foods designed to look and taste like meat. Most are made of soybeans but some contain wheat, peanuts, yeast, and eggs. Many have a long list of additives and may be quite high in sodium.

COMPLEMENT YOUR PROTEIN

The six categories shown represent alternate protein foods. To make them high-quality protein, equal to meat, combine any food from one column with any food from another column *at the same meal.* Example: **whole-wheat bread + peanut butter or brown rice + lentils. This is called "protein complementation."**

Grains	*Legumes*	*Dairy Foods*	*Eggs*	*Nuts*	*Seeds*
Barley	Black beans	Cheese	Any style	Almonds	Pumpkin seeds
Brown rice	Blackeyed peas	cottage		Brazil nuts	Sesame seeds
Buckwheat (kasha)	Chickpeas	natural		Cashew nuts	Sesame butter
Bulgur	(garbanzos)	processed		Chestnuts	(tahini)
Cornmeal	Kidney beans	Dry milk products		Coconut	Squash seeds
Cracked wheat	Lentils	Milk		Hazel nuts	Sunflower seeds
Millet	Lima beans	Yogurt		Pecans	
Noodles	Mung beans			Pine nuts	
Oatmeal	Mung bean sprouts			Pistachio nuts	
Pasta	Navy beans			Walnuts	
Rice	Pea beans				
Rye	Peanuts				
Wheat berries	Peanut butter				
Wheat germ	Peas				
Whole wheat	Pinto beans				
	Soybeans				
	Soybean sprouts				
	Soy flour				
	Soy protein				
	Soy milk				
	Split peas				
	Tofu (soybean curd)				

As meat prices rise and consumers desire to cut their intake of saturated fats and cholesterol, *meat analogs* are being used more. Imitation bacon and sausages have not become as popular as manufacturers had hoped because meat flavor duplication is somewhat disappointing. One meat analog, though, has become a supermarket and salad bar staple: BacOs, imitation bacon bits, marketed by General Mills, are actually spun soybean.

* What is tofu?

Pronounced "toe-foo," this unusual food is sold as white pillows or pads, about three inches square, submerged in water and resembling bars of soap. What is it? A low-calorie, no-cholesterol plant protein. Tofu, also called "bean curd" or "soy cheese," is soy milk compressed into square cakes resembling farmer's cheese. The only addition is calcium sulfate, used as a solidifier.

Chinese, Japanese, and Koreans have used it for centuries. We have only caught on to its versatility lately. Specialty food shops and supermarkets in Chinatown always carried tofu. Today you may find it at your local dairy store or grocery. Here it will be sold packed in plastic containers and found in the dairy case or with the fresh vegetables.

Tofu may be eaten hot, cold, cooked, or uncooked. Bland by itself, it absorbs flavors and resembles the tender white meat of chicken when cooked. Mashed or blended, it can replace cream or sour cream as a natural thickener. Naturally low in fat and calories and free of cholesterol, tofu provides protein, calcium, phosphorus, potassium, and some B vitamins and E.

It's a food you'll enjoy experimenting with since it can be prepared in so many ways. An Oriental or vegetarian cookbook will provide numerous ideas. Mixed one to one with peanut butter it makes a fluffy spread with added protein and reduced fat and calories. Try our Tofu Stir-Fry in the recipe section of this chapter.

* I can't imagine not eating meat. What would you eat?

Vegetarian or not, all of us frequently eat nonmeat meals—a breakfast of cereal, toast, coffee, and juice; perhaps pizza at lunch; or eggplant parmigiana for dinner. Often, unknowingly, we go a few days without eating meat and never miss it. You can too with a little imagination. If you are adding fiber to your diet, eating more fresh fruits and vegetables, and cutting down on fat you will also be cutting down on meat.

Just to show you it can be done, we've included a seven-day menu excluding meat, fish, and poultry. See "One-Week Vegetarian Menu" section in this chapter. The meals are balanced, appealing, tasty, and nutritious. See what you think.

ONE-WEEK VEGETARIAN MENU

MONDAY

Breakfast
Orange juice
Oatmeal
Whole-wheat toast
Coffee, tea, skim milk

Lunch
Pita bread pocket filled
 with Bean Dip* and
 shredded lettuce
Fresh vegetables cut up
 (cauliflower, mushrooms,
 carrots, celery)
Brownie
Skim milk

Dinner
Macaroni and cheese
Waldorf salad
Rice Muffin†
Fresh fruit cup
Beverage of choice

TUESDAY

Breakfast
Sliced strawberries
French toast with syrup
Coffee, tea, skim milk

* See The Recipes Section in This Chapter.
† See The Special Muffin Recipes in Chapter 1.

TUESDAY (cont.)

Lunch
The Best Ever Split Pea Soup*
Cheese and crackers
Grapes
Oatmeal cookies
Skim milk

Dinner
Tofu-Stir Fry* over brown rice
Sesame seed bread sticks
Spinach salad
Ice cream and cookies
Beverage of choice

WEDNESDAY

Breakfast
Grapefruit half
Raisin Bran
Whole-wheat English muffin
Coffee, tea, skim milk

Lunch
Pizza
Tossed salad
Fresh melon
Skim milk

Dinner
Hearty Bean-Vegetable Soup*
Pumpernickel bread
Lettuce wedge and choice of
  dressing
Rice pudding
Beverage of choice

THURSDAY

Breakfast
Stewed fruit
Scrambled egg
Corn Muffin†
Coffee, tea, skim milk

Lunch
Grilled Swiss cheese and
  tomato on whole-wheat
  bread
Three-bean salad
Pear
Skim milk

Dinner
Baked potato topped with
  mixed vegetables in
  cream sauce
Corn on the cob
Broccoli with garlic and lemon
Carrot-raisin salad
Pound cake
Beverage of choice

FRIDAY

Breakfast
Grapefruit juice
Wheatena
Rye toast with jelly
Coffee, tea, skim milk

Lunch
Egg salad sandwich
Red cabbage slaw
Raisins and nuts
Fresh apple
Skim milk

FRIDAY (cont.)

Dinner
Country Cheese Pie*
Stewed tomatoes
Fresh green beans
Tossed salad
Apple Muffin†
Blueberry cobbler
Beverage of choice

SATURDAY

Breakfast
Banana
Cold cereal
Whole-wheat toast
Coffee, tea, skim milk

Lunch
Cream of Carrot Soup*
Chef's salad with hard-boiled
  egg
Oatmeal-Yogurt Muffin†
Date cookies
Skim milk

Dinner
Eggplant parmigiana
Italian salad
Whole-wheat Italian bread
Sherbet
Beverage of choice

SUNDAY

Breakfast
Fruit-topped yogurt
Bran Muffin†
Coffee, tea, skim milk

Lunch
Mushroom omelet
Marinated vegetable salad
Corn bread
Apple crisp
Skim milk

Dinner
Crunchy Vegetable-Rice Dinner*
Lettuce wedge and choice of
  dressing
Seeded bread sticks
Banana bread
Beverage of choice

* See The Recipes Section in This Chapter.
† See The Special Muffin Recipes in Chapter 1.

* Since I began eating vegetarian meals the palms of my hands have yellowed. Is this dangerous?

This is a harmless condition called "carotenemia." You are probably eating large amounts of deep yellow-orange and dark green leafy vegetables and fruits (i.e., carrots, squash, broccoli, spinach, kale, apricots, peaches). These are high in carotene, a substance that can be converted to vitamin A in your body. In your case, you are eating more carotene than your body is converting. Carotene is accumulating, giving your skin a yellowish cast. It is most predominant on the soles of the feet and palms of the hands.

Carotenemia often results when the enthusiastic new owner of a juicer begins guzzling carrot juice. High amounts of carotene may be drunk and will quickly begin yellowing the skin. Yellowing may also result from jaundice, a symptom of liver disease. In this case, the whites of the eyes yellow as well; in carotenemia they do not.

To prevent further yellowing (though harmless) or to get rid of the yellow tinge, limit your carotene-containing foods to one a day. In two to six weeks your color should return to normal. See Chapter 2's charts "Vitamin Sources" and "Vitamin A Content of Some Foods" for a list of foods high in vitamin A. The fruits and vegetables on this list are high in carotene and are the ones to limit, if you wish.

* What are macrobiotic foods?

Zen macrobiotic is a type of vegetarian diet with an elaborate system of balancing foods based on the characteristics the foods are believed to have. Macrobiotics means the path to longevity and peace of mind through belief in Zen and the adoption of rigid dietary practices. There is extensive food avoidance, especially during illness, and fluids may be withheld as well. No foods are "macrobiotic" but some foods are closely associated with this eating pattern—tamari (fermented soy sauce), miso (soybean paste), gomasio (sesame seed salt), umeboshi (salted plums), and various seaweeds.

Macrobiotic believers feel no disease is incurable and diet can provide physical, mental, and spiritual purification.

In a series of ten diet plans ranging from minus three to seven, diet seven is regarded as the one with the greatest curative properties. It is 100 percent cereal with the major food being brown rice. The only other item allowed is water, and it is suggested that it be taken "sparingly." The sicker a person becomes the more he is encouraged to stay on an all-brown rice diet alternating with fasting. The promised results are wellness and euphoria. The actual results have been the disorientation associated with starvation and in some cases death.

Even though diet plans minus one, two, and three are more liberal, they still do not provide good nutrition. Macrobiotic followers have suffered serious nutritional deficiencies such as scurvy (lack of vitamin C), rickets (lack of vitamin D), anemia (lack of iron), hypocalcemia (low serum calcium), malnutrition, and loss of kidney function caused by the restricted fluids.

It would seem that no one in his right mind would voluntarily follow this diet pattern, but many have. In the pursuit of health and long life people often are misled into bizarre lifestyles. Be cautious of any diet plan that makes promises for eternal life, health, or happiness.

* Is fasting a good way to rid my body of poisons?

You are told to fast to rest the digestive tract, to rid yourself of poisons, to remove excess acid production from bodily organs, or to lose weight rapidly. All suggest a purification, a cleansing, and a fresh start with a revitalized body. In fact your body and your digestive tract never rest and they do not need to. Even while you sleep, your cells and organs are hard at work. The work you do during waking hours, that which you are aware of, accounts for only about one-third of the work or total energy you spend in a day.

The body's top priority is to burn energy to meet its needs. To do this efficiently you need periodic refueling—in short, eating regularly.

When you fast, you remove your primary source of fuel and the body must look for an alternate. It does not shut down and wait till the fast is over. If you are starving, there is no food. If you are fasting, you choose not to eat. The result is the same, your body is forced to use its own reserves for fuel. Its stored carbohydrate is exhausted in hours and then fat and muscle breakdown begins. Simultaneously, the body shifts into low gear, drastically reducing its energy needs to conserve itself. Otherwise body loss would be so rapid it would be fatal.

The result of all this is that body functions are not efficient. The liver and kidney, which clear toxic substances, are not working normally. Acid production is mounting due to the wastes of muscle breakdown and incomplete fat breakdown. Believe it or not, fat loss is slower than the loss that would occur on a low-calorie diet. Fasting for a few hours or up to a full day probably will leave you hungry and irritable but will do no harm. Extended fasting, however, has no benefit and may cause serious problems.

RECIPES

* Where can I find vegetarian recipes?

Almost all cookbooks feature recipes with cheese, rice, beans, or pasta as main dishes. Ethnic or cultural cookbooks are especially interesting sources. Look over the cookbook section in your local bookstore; the selection of vegetarian cookbooks is expanding. Two that we particularly enjoy using are:

Laurel's Kitchen: A Handbook for Vegetarian Cookery and Nutrition by Laurel Robertson, Carol Flinders, and Bronwen Godfrey, Bantam Books. (Originally published by Nilgiri Press, Petaluma, California 94853, 1976.)

Moosewood Cookbook by Mollie Katzen, Ten Speed Press, P. O. Box 7123, Berkeley, California 94707, 1977.

Following are a small collection of nonmeat recipes we cook and enjoy. We hope you will too.

The Best Ever Split Pea Soup

Makes 12 servings (approximately 1 cup each)

1 pound split peas
10 cups water
½ pound carrots, pared and cut in large pieces
½ pound (about 3) parsnips, cut in large pieces
2 medium onions, peeled and quartered

Rinse split peas thoroughly and sort; place in a large pot and cover with water. Bring to a boil, boil 2 minutes, turn off heat, and let split peas soak 1 hour; drain.

Add 10 cups water to the peas; bring to a boil, reduce to simmer, and cook over medium heat for ½ hour.

Add carrots, parsnips, and onion; continue cooking 1 hour or until split peas are tender.

HINT: For variety, 1 pound of yellow split peas may be substituted for 1 pound green split peas.

NOTE: This recipe may be cut in half if you wish to make a smaller amount. We prefer to make a large pot of soup and freeze half for future use. This soup may be frozen for up to six months without loss of flavor or quality.

1 cup (8 ounces) soup contains 209 calories, 34 mg. sodium

Cream of Carrot Soup

Makes 8 servings (approximately 1 cup each)

4 cups water
1½ pounds of carrots, pared and cut in large pieces
3 medium potatoes, pared and cut in large pieces
2 stalks celery, sliced
3 cloves garlic, chopped
1 cup chopped onion
3 tablespoons unsalted butter or margarine*
1 cup skim milk

In a large saucepan bring water to a boil; add carrots, potatoes, and celery; cover and simmer 15 minutes.

While vegetables cook, sauté garlic and onion in butter until clear and soft, about 5 minutes.

Do not drain cooked vegetables. Place vegetables, cooking liquid, and sautéed onion in a blender container and puree until smooth. Return puree to saucepan.

Add skim milk; warm and serve.

NOTE: This recipe may be cut in half if you wish to make a smaller amount. We prefer to make a large pot of soup and freeze half for future use. This soup may be frozen for up to three months without loss of flavor or quality.
1 cup (8 ounces) soup contains 116 calories, 119 mg. sodium, *68 mg. sodium

Hearty Bean-Vegetable Soup
Makes 6 servings (approximately 1 cup each)

1 cup navy beans
3 cups water
1 16-ounce can tomato puree
1 cup sliced anise or celery
2 tablespoons chopped fresh parsley
½ cup chopped onion
3 carrots, sliced in coins
½ cup elbow macaroni, uncooked
6 escarole leaves, washed and cut in large pieces

Cover beans with water in a large kettle; bring to a boil, boil 2 minutes, turn off heat, and let stand 1 hour; drain beans.

Return beans to kettle and add 3 cups water; bring to a boil, cover, reduce to simmer, and cook 1½ hours.

Add tomato puree, anise, parsley, onion, and carrots; cover and cook 30 minutes.

Add elbow macaroni; cover and cook 15 minutes.

Add escarole; cover and cook 2 to 5 minutes or until escarole is wilted. Soup will be quite thick. It may be thinned with water, if you wish.

HINT: Individual servings may be seasoned with a sprinkle of fresh ground pepper or a dash of cayenne pepper or cumin.
1 serving (1 cup): 207 calories, 360 mg. sodium

Bean Dip
Makes approximately 2⅔ cups

3 cups cooked kidney beans
1 medium onion, finely chopped (½ cup)
2 cloves garlic, crushed
1 tablespoon oil
½ teaspoon dry coriander (optional)
½ teaspoon dill
⅛ teaspoon pepper
1 cup walnuts, finely chopped

Mash beans to a very smooth puree.

Sauté onions and garlic in oil until soft, about 5 minutes.

Thoroughly combine beans, sautéed onion, and remaining ingredients.

> NOTE: This recipe makes a nice dip with raw vegetables or it can be used as a spread on toast or filling for pita bread pockets.
>
> 1 serving (⅓ cup) contains 200 calories, 4 mg. sodium

Country Cheese Pie
Makes 8 servings

1 cup oatmeal
1 cup shredded cheddar cheese (about 4 oz.)
½ to 1 teaspoon dry mustard
2 eggs
½ cup skim milk
1 frozen prepared piecrust (homemade may be used as well)

Coarsely grind oatmeal in a blender for about 15 seconds.

Combine oatmeal, cheese, mustard, and eggs.

Put mixture into a piecrust and bake at 350°F for 30 minutes.

> NOTE: This recipe makes a nice change for breakfast or as a main dish served with a salad and a vegetable. A homemade piecrust made without added salt will lower the sodium content by approximately 45 percent to 121 mg. sodium per serving.
>
> Per serving: 203 calories, 224 mg. sodium

Tofu Stir-Fry

Makes 4 servings or 6 when served with brown rice

2 tablespoons oil
1 large onion chopped (1 cup)
2 cloves garlic
2 tofu (soybean curd) cakes (2½″ × 2¾″ × 1″)
¼ cup walnuts, coarsely chopped
½ pound mushrooms, washed and sliced
2 medium zucchini, washed and sliced in coins (about 2 cups)
1 green pepper, seeded and sliced
1 cup frozen peas
½ teaspoon sesame seed oil
1 teaspoon soy sauce
2 teaspoons molasses
1 cup fresh bean sprouts

Heat oil in a large skillet; sauté onion and garlic till soft.

Slice tofu cakes in ¼-inch slices (domino-shaped pieces); place in skillet in a single layer; let brown lightly and gently turn with pancake turner to brown other side; add walnuts.

Add mushrooms, zucchini, pepper, and peas; sauté 5 to 7 minutes, until vegetables are crisp-tender.

Add sesame seed oil, soy sauce, and molasses; stir to combine.

Add bean sprouts, cover skillet, and let stand 3 to 5 minutes; serve plain or over cooked brown rice.

1 serving (plain) contains 211 calories, 174 mg. sodium
1 serving with ½ cup brown rice: 218 calories, 122 mg. sodium

Crunchy Vegetable-Rice Dinner

Makes 6 servings

½ cup brown rice
½ head broccoli (about 2 cups)
½ head cauliflower (about 2 cups)
2 tablespoons oil
4 to 6 cloves garlic, diced
1 medium carrot, pared and thinly sliced
1 small summer squash, washed and diced (about 1 cup)
½ red pepper, thinly sliced
4 ounces cheddar cheese, sliced
4 ounces muenster or Swiss cheese, sliced

Cook brown rice, following package directions, omitting salt; set aside.

While rice is cooking cut broccoli and cauliflower in small flowerets and dice stems.

Heat oil in a medium-size frying pan; add garlic and brown; add broccoli, cauliflower, carrot, and squash; stir-fry over medium-hight heat about 10 minutes or until vegetables are crisp-tender. It is important to stir frequently to prevent burning and sticking.

In a 9″ × 13″ shallow baking dish layer rice, then stir-fried vegetables, and remaining pan oil and fried vegetable bits; add red pepper slices and top with alternating slices of the two cheeses.

Bake at 350°F for 20 to 25 minutes.

> HINT: Almost all the sodium in this recipe is contributed by the two cheeses. If you use no-salt or low-salt varieties of cheese you will reduce the sodium a great deal.
>
> NOTE: This recipe can be made a day ahead and heated for serving. It can also be doubled for a party or a crowd.
>
> 1 serving (approximately 1½ cups): 277 calories, 281 mg. sodium

APPENDIX

Fast Foods

Fast food restaurants flank American highways today like the Burma Shave signs of long ago. There isn't a state in the union that doesn't have at least one set of Golden Arches (McDonald's). Over 98 percent of all Americans recognize that symbol and almost as many have eaten a Big Mac.

Fast foods are usually associated with the youth and speed of the younger generation. Nothing could be further from the truth. The founder of fast foods, Colonel Sanders, was sixty-two when he began selling franchises for his Kentucky Fried Chicken in the early 1950s. Every week 52 percent of all fast food meals are eaten by those over age forty. Fast foods are part of the American way of eating and they are here to stay. We need to look more closely at the contribution these foods are making to our nutritional well-being. Interestingly, when people eat in a fast food restaurant, nutrition is not the foremost concern. Customers rank freshness and price as primary concerns, with nutrition running in third place.

Fast foods have been accused of offering little nutrition. This is not so. A fast food meal supplies substantial protein as well as B vitamins, iron, and calcium. The chief problem is caloric density— the typical meal averages over 1,000 calories and is high in fat and sodium. Calories can be lowered if a plain hamburger is substituted for one with "all the trimmings," a salad is chosen with a small amount of dressing instead of french fries, and milk replaces the shake. Sodium content is harder for the customer to control. A fast food meal may contain over 2,500 milligrams of sodium with the entrees contributing the largest amount. Those who must choose a low-sodium diet will find their selections limited. Seafood or steak restaurants might allow more flexibility since items may be broiled to order.

Eating at a fast food restaurant requires some nutrition knowledge so that wise choices can be made. Franchises are changing their menu items, offering unbreaded, broiled fish; items cooked without salt; salad; bread; and fresh fruit bars all of which provide more variety and better nutrition. The following "Analyses of Fast Foods" gives a calorie and nutrient breakdown of some representative menu items. Look it over so that you will be a more educated consumer the next time you drive through those "golden arches."

NOTE: Adapted from "Perspective on Fast Foods," *Dietetic Currents,* E. A. Young, Ross Laboratories, Columbus, Ohio, 1981; and *Food Values of Portions Commonly Used,* 13th ed. J. A. T. Pennington and H. N. Church, Harper & Row Publishers, 1980.

Nutritional Analyses of Fast Foods

(Dashes indicate no data available. X = Less than 2 % US RDA; tr=trace.)

	Wt (g)	Energy (kcal)	PRO (g)	CHO (g)	Fat (g)	Chol (mg)	Vitamins A (IU)	B_1 (mg)	B_2 (mg)	Nia. (mg)	B_6 (mg)	B_{12} (µg)	C (mg)	D (IU)	Minerals Ca (mg)	Cu (mg)	Fe (mg)	K (mg)	Mg (mg)	P (mg)	Na (mg)	Zn (mg)	Mois-ture (g)	Crude Fiber (g)
ARBY'S																								
Roast Beef	140	350	22	32	15	45	X	0.30	0.34	5	–	–	X	–	80	–	3.6	–	–	–	880	–	–	–
Beef and Cheese	168	450	27	36	22	55	X	0.38	0.43	6	–	–	X	–	200	–	4.5	–	–	–	1220	–	–	–
Super Roast Beef	263	620	30	61	28	85	X	0.53	0.43	7	–	–	X	–	100	–	5.4	–	–	–	1420	–	–	–
Junior Roast Beef	74	220	12	21	9	35	X	0.15	0.17	3	–	–	X	–	40	–	1.8	–	–	–	530	–	–	–
Ham & Cheese	154	380	28	33	17	60	X	0.75	0.34	5	–	–	X	–	200	–	2.7	–	–	–	1350	–	–	–
Turkey Deluxe	236	510	28	46	24	70	X	0.45	0.34	8	–	–	X	–	80	–	2.7	–	–	–	1220	–	–	–
Club Sandwich	252	560	30	43	30	100	X	0.68	0.43	7	–	–	X	–	200	–	3.6	–	–	–	1610	–	–	–

Source: Consumer Affairs, Arby's, Inc, Atlanta, Georgia. Nutritional analysis by Technological Resources, Camden, New Jersey

	Wt (g)	Energy (kcal)	PRO (g)	CHO (g)	Fat (g)	Chol (mg)	A (IU)	B_1 (mg)	B_2 (mg)	Nia. (mg)	B_6 (mg)	B_{12} (µg)	C (mg)	D (IU)	Ca (mg)	Cu (mg)	Fe (mg)	K (mg)	Mg (mg)	P (mg)	Na (mg)	Zn (mg)	Mois-ture (g)	Crude Fiber (g)
BURGER CHEF																								
Hamburger	91	244	11	29	9	27	114	0.17	0.16	2.7	0.16	0.26	1.2	–	45	0.08	2.0	208	9	106	–	1.6	41	0.2
Cheeseburger	104	290	14	29	13	39	267	0.18	0.21	2.8	0.17	0.36	1.2	–	132	0.08	2.2	218	9	202	–	1.9	46	0.2
Double Cheeseburger	145	420	24	30	22	77	431	0.20	0.32	4.4	0.31	0.73	1.2	–	223	0.10	3.2	360	15	355	–	3.6	67	0.2
Fish Filet	179	547	21	46	31	43	400	0.23	0.22	2.7	0.04	0.10	1.0	–	145	0.04	2.2	271	19	302	–	1.2	72	0.4
Super Shef* Sandwich	252	563	29	44	30	105	754	0.31	0.40	6.0	0.45	0.87	9.3	–	205	0.21	4.5	578	25	377	–	4.5	143	0.5
Big Shef* Sandwich	186	569	23	38	36	81	279	0.26	0.31	4.7	0.31	0.63	1.0	–	152	0.05	3.6	382	14	280	–	3.4	80	0.3
TOP Shef* Sandwich	138	661	41	36	38	134	273	0.35	0.47	8.1	0.56	1.16	0	–	194	0.13	5.4	612	26	445	–	5.9	91	0.1
Funmeal* Feast	–	545	15	55	30	27	123	0.25	0.21	4.6	0.16	0.26	12.8	–	61	0.24	2.8	688	26	183	–	1.6	70	0.8
Rancher® Platter*	316	640	32	33	42	106	1750*	0.29	0.38	8.6	0.61	1.01	23.5	–	66	0.38	5.3	1237	53	326	–	5.6	209	1.3
Mariner® Platter*	373	734	29	78	34	35	2069*	0.34	0.23	5.2	0.09	0.56	23.5	–	63	0.32	3.3	996	49	397	–	1.2	195	1.8
French Fries, small	68	250	2	20	19	0	0	0.07	0.04	1.7	–	0	11.5	–	9	0.16	0.7	473	16	62	–	<0.1	29	0.6
French Fries, large	85	351	3	28	26	0	0	0.10	0.06	2.4	–	0	16.2	–	13	0.23	0.9	661	22	86	–	<0.1	40	0.9
Vanilla Shake (12 oz)	336	380	13	60	10	40	387	0.10	0.66	0.5	0.1	1.77	0	–	497	–	0.3	622	40	392	–	1.3	–	–
Chocolate Shake (12 oz)	336	403	10	72	9	36	292	0.16	0.76	0.4	0.1	1.07	0	–	449	–	1.1	762	54	429	–	1.6	–	–
Hot Chocolate	–	198	8	23	8	30	288	0.93	0.39	0.3	0.1	0.79	2.1	–	271	0.09	0.7	436	50	245	–	1.1	–	–

*Includes salad Source Burger Chef Systems, Inc, Indianapolis, Indiana Nutritional analysis from Handbook No. 8 Washington US Dept of Agriculture

	Wt (g)	Energy (kcal)	PRO (g)	CHO (g)	Fat (g)	Chol (mg)	A (IU)	B_1 (mg)	B_2 (mg)	Nia. (mg)	B_6 (mg)	B_{12} (µg)	C (mg)	D (IU)	Ca (mg)	Cu (mg)	Fe (mg)	K (mg)	Mg (mg)	P (mg)	Na (mg)	Zn (mg)	Mois-ture (g)	Crude Fiber (g)
CHURCH'S FRIED CHICKEN																								
White Chicken Portion	100	327	21	10	23	–	160	0.10	0.18	7.2	–	–	0.7	–	94	–	1.00	186	–	–	498	–	45	0.10
Dark Chicken Portion	100	305	22	7	21	–	140	0.10	0.27	5.3	–	–	1.0	–	15	–	1.3	206	–	–	475	–	48	0.20

Source: Church's Fried Chicken, San Antonio, Texas, Nutritional analysis by Medallion Laboratories, Minneapolis, Minnesota

Nutritional Analyses of Fast Foods

(Dashes indicate no data available. X = Less than 2% US RDA; tr=trace.)

							Vitamins								Minerals									
	Wt (g)	Energy (kcal)	PRO (g)	CHO (g)	Fat (g)	Chol (mg)	A (IU)	B_1 (mg)	B_2 (mg)	Nia. (mg)	B_6 (mg)	B_{12} (µg)	C (mg)	D (IU)	Ca (mg)	Cu (mg)	Fe (mg)	K (mg)	Mg (mg)	P (mg)	Na (mg)	Zn (mg)	Mois-ture (g)	Crude Fiber (g)
DAIRY QUEEN®																								
Frozen Dessert	113	180	5	27	6	20	100	0.09	0.17	X	–	0.6	X	X	150	0.08	X	–	–	100	–	–	–	–
DQ Cone, small	71	110	3	18	3	10	100	0.03	0.14	X	–	0.4	X	X	100	–	X	–	–	60	–	–	–	–
DQ Cone, regular	142	230	6	35	7	10	300	0.09	0.26	X	–	0.6	X	X	200	–	X	–	–	150	–	–	–	–
DQ Cone, large	213	340	10	52	10	30	400	0.15	0.43	X	–	1.2	X	8	300	–	X	–	–	200	–	–	–	–
DQ Dip Cone, small	78	150	3	20	7	10	100	0.03	0.17	X	–	0.4	X	X	100	–	X	–	–	80	–	–	–	–
DQ Dip Cone, regular	156	300	7	40	13	20	300	0.09	0.34	X	–	0.6	X	8	200	–	0.4	–	–	150	–	–	–	–
DQ Dip Cone, large	234	450	10	58	20	30	400	0.12	0.51	X	–	0.9	X	8	300	–	0.7	–	–	100	–	–	–	–
DQ Sundae, small	106	170	4	30	4	15	100	0.03	0.17	0.4	–	0.5	X	X	100	–	–	–	–	100	–	–	–	–
DQ Sundae, regular	177	290	6	51	7	20	300	0.06	0.26	0.4	–	0.6	X	X	200	–	1.1	–	–	150	–	–	–	–
DQ Sundae, large	248	400	9	71	9	30	400	0.09	0.43	0.8	–	1.2	X	8	300	–	1.1	–	–	250	–	–	–	–
DQ Malt, small	241	340	10	51	11	30	400	0.06	0.34	0.8	–	1.2	2.4	8	500	–	1.8	–	–	200	–	–	–	–
DQ Malt, regular	418	600	15	89	20	50	750	0.12	0.60	0.8	–	1.8	3.6	60	600	–	3.6	–	–	600	–	–	–	–
DQ Malt, large	588	840	22	125	28	70	750	0.15	0.85	1.2	–	2.4	6	100	600	–	5.4	–	–	200	–	–	–	–
DQ Float	397	330	6	59	8	20	100	0.12	0.17	X	–	0.6	X	140	200	–	–	–	–	250	–	–	–	–
DQ Banana Split	383	540	10	91	15	30	750	0.60	0.60	0.8	–	0.9	18	X	350	–	1.8	–	–	250	–	–	–	–
DQ Parfait	284	460	10	81	11	30	400	0.12	0.43	0.4	–	1.2	X	8	300	–	1.8	–	–	250	–	–	–	–
DQ Freeze	397	520	11	89	13	35	200	0.15	0.34	X	–	1.2	X	X	300	–	–	–	–	200	–	–	–	–
Mr. Misty* Freeze	411	500	10	87	12	20	200	0.12	0.17	X	–	0.12	X	X	300	–	X	–	–	200	–	–	–	–
Mr. Misty* Float	404	440	6	85	8	20	100	0.06	0.17	X	–	0.6	X	X	200	–	X	–	–	100	–	–	–	–
"Dilly"* Bar	85	240	4	22	15	10	100	0.03	0.17	0.4	–	0.5	X	X	100	–	0.4	–	–	60	–	–	–	–
DQ Sandwich	60	140	3	24	4	10	100	X	0.14	X	–	0.2	X	X	60	–	0.4	–	–	X	–	–	–	–
Mr. Misty Kiss*	89	70	0	17	0	0	X	X	X	X	–	X	X	X	X	–	X	–	–	–	–	–	–	–
Brazier* Cheese Dog	113	330	15	24	19	–	–	–	0.18	3.3	0.07	1.22	11.0	23	168	0.08	1.6	–	24	182	939	1.9	–	–
Brazier* Chili Dog	128	330	13	25	20	–	–	0.15	0.23	3.9	0.17	1.05	11.0	20	86	0.13	2.0	–	38	139	868	1.8	–	–
Brazier* Dog	99	273	11	23	15	–	–	0.12	0.15	2.6	0.08	1.05	tr	23	75	0.09	1.5	–	21	104	–	1.4	–	–
Fish Sandwich	170	400	20	41	17	–	100	0.15	0.26	3.0	0.16	1.20	tr	40	60	0.08	1.1	–	24	200	1552	0.3	–	–
Fish Sandwich w/Ch	177	440	24	39	21	–	tr	0.15	0.44	3.0	0.16	1.50	14.0	40	150	0.08	0.4	–	37	250	–	0.3	–	–
Super Brazier* Dog	182	518	20	41	30	–	tr	0.42	0.48	7.0	0.17	2.09	14.0	44	158	0.18	4.3	–	42	195	1986	2.8	–	–
Super Brazier* Dog w/Ch	203	593	26	43	36	–	tr	0.43	0.48	8.1	0.18	2.34	14.0	44	297	0.21	4.4	–	48	312	–	3.5	–	–
Super Brazier* Chili Dog	210	555	23	42	33	–	tr	0.42	0.48	8.8	0.27	2.67	18.0	32	158	–	4.0	–	–	231	1640	2.8	–	–
Brazier* Fries, small	71	200	2	25	10	–	tr	0.06	tr	0.8	0.16	–	3.6	16	tr	0.04	0.4	–	16	100	–	tr	–	–
Brazier* Fries, large	113	320	3	40	16	–	tr	0.09	0.03	1.2	0.30	–	4.8	24	tr	0.08	0.4	–	24	150	–	0.3	–	–
Brazier* Onion Rings	85	300	6	33	17	–	tr	0.09	–	0.4	0.08	X	2.4	32	20	0.08	0.4	–	16	60	–	0.3	–	–

Source: International Dairy Queen, Inc. Minneapolis, Minnesota. Nutritional analysis by Raltech Scientific Services, Inc. (formerly WARF), Madison, Wisconsin. (Nutritional analysis not applicable in the state of Texas.)

298

JACK IN THE BOX®

Hamburger	97	263	13	29	11	26	49	0.27	0.18	5.6	0.11	0.73	1.1	20	82	0.10	2.3	165	20	115	566	1.8	43	0.2
Cheeseburger	109	310	16	28	15	32	338	0.27	0.21	5.4	0.12	0.87	<1.1	20	172	0.10	2.6	177	22	194	877	2.3	47	0.2
Jumbo Jack® Hamburger	246	551	28	45	29	80	246	0.47	0.34	11.6	0.30	2.68	3.7	42	134	0.22	4.5	492	44	261	1134	4.2	139	0.7
Jumbo Jack® Hamburger w/Ch	272	628	32	45	35	110	734	0.52	0.38	11.3	0.31	3.05	4.9	41	273	0.24	4.6	499	49	411	1666	4.8	153	0.8
Regular Taco	83	189	8	15	11	22	356	0.07	0.08	1.8	0.14	0.5	<0.9	6	116	0.11	1.2	264	36	150	460	1.3	47	0.6
Super Taco	146	285	12	20	17	37	599	0.10	0.12	2.8	0.22	0.77	1.6	9	196	0.18	1.9	415	53	235	968	2.1	92	1.0
Moby Jack® Sandwich	141	455	17	38	26	56	240	0.30	0.21	4.5	0.12	1.1	1.4	24	167	0.08	1.7	246	30	263	837	1.1	57	0.1
Breakfast Jack® Sandwich	121	301	18	28	13	182	442	0.41	0.47	5.1	0.14	1.1	3.4	51	177	0.11	2.5	190	24	310	1037	1.8	59	0.1
French Fries	80	270	3	31	15	13	-	0.12	0.02	1.9	0.22	0.17	3.7	<1	19	0.10	0.7	423	27	88	128	0.3	29	0.6
Onion Rings	85	351	5	32	23	24	-	0.24	0.12	3.1	0.07	0.26	<1.2	<1	26	0.07	1.4	109	16	69	318	0.4	24	0.3
Apple Turnover	119	411	4	45	24	17	-	0.23	0.12	2.5	0.03	0.17	<1.2	1	11	0.06	1.4	69	10	33	352	0.2	45	0.2
Vanilla Shake*	317	317	10	57	6	26	-	0.16	0.38	0.5	0.20	1.36	<3.2	41	349	0.06	0.2	599	38	312	229	1.0	243	0.3
Strawberry Shake*	328	323	11	55	7	26	-	0.16	0.46	0.6	0.15	1.25	<3.3	43	371	0.10	0.6	613	40	328	241	1.1	253	0.3
Chocolate Shake*	322	325	11	55	7	26	-	0.16	0.64	0.6	0.19	1.55	<3.2	45	348	0.13	0.7	676	53	328	270	1.1	247	0.3
Vanilla Shake	314	342	10	54	9	36	440	0.16	0.47	0.5	0.18	1.1	3.5	44	349	0.06	0.4	536	48	318	263	1.0	238	0.3
Strawberry Shake	328	380	11	63	10	33	426	0.16	0.62	0.5	0.18	0.92	<3.3	30	351	0.07	0.3	556	47	316	268	1.0	242	0.3
Chocolate Shake	317	365	11	59	10	35	380	0.16	0.60	0.6	0.18	0.98	<3.2	38	350	0.16	1.2	633	57	332	294	1.2	235	0.3
Ham & Cheese Omelette	174	425	21	32	23	355	766	0.45	0.70	3.0	0.18	1.44	<1.7	64	260	0.14	4.0	237	29	397	975	2.3	94	0.2
Double Cheese Omelette	166	423	19	30	25	370	797	0.33	0.68	2.5	0.14	1.33	1.7	61	276	0.13	3.6	208	26	370	899	2.1	88	0.2
Ranchero Style Omelette	196	414	20	33	23	343	853	0.33	0.74	2.6	0.18	1.51	<2.0	78	278	0.14	3.8	260	29	372	1098	2.0	117	0.4
French Toast	180	537	15	54	29	115	522	0.56	0.30	4.4	0.47	1.62	9.2	22	119	0.11	3.0	194	27	256	1130	1.8	78	0.9
Pancakes	232	626	16	79	27	87	488	0.63	0.44	4.6	0.19	0.56	<26.2	23	105	0.12	2.8	237	36	633	1670	1.9	104	0.7
Scrambled Eggs	267	719	26	55	44	259	694	0.69	0.56	5.2	0.34	1.31	<12.8	80	257	0.24	5.0	635	55	483	1110	3.0	137	1.3

*Special formula for shakes sold in California, Arizona, Texas and Washington. Source: Jack-in-the-Box, Foodmaker, Inc. San Diego, California. Nutritional analysis by Raltech Scientific Services, Inc. (formerly WARF), Madison, Wisconsin.

KENTUCKY FRIED CHICKEN®

Original Recipe® Dinner*

Wing & Rib	322	603	30	48	32	133	25.5	0.22	0.19	10.0	-	-	36.6	-	-	-	-	-	-	-	-	-	-	-
Wing & Thigh	341	661	33	48	38	172	25.5	0.24	0.27	8.4	-	-	36.6	-	-	-	-	-	-	-	-	-	-	-
Drum & Thigh	346	643	35	46	35	180	25.5	0.25	0.32	8.5	-	-	36.6	-	-	-	-	-	-	-	-	-	-	-

Extra Crispy Dinner*

Wing & Rib	349	755	33	60	43	132	25.5	0.31	0.29	10.4	-	-	36.6	-	-	-	-	-	-	-	-	-	-	-
Wing & Thigh	371	812	36	58	48	176	25.5	0.31	0.35	10.3	-	-	36.6	-	-	-	-	-	-	-	-	-	-	-
Drum & Thigh	376	765	38	55	44	183	25.5	0.32	0.38	10.4	-	-	36.6	-	-	-	-	-	-	-	-	-	-	-
Mashed Potatoes	85	64	2	12	1	0	<18	<0.01	0.02	0.8	-	-	4.9	-	-	-	-	-	-	-	-	-	-	-
Gravy	14	23	0	1	2	0	<3	0.00	0.01	0.1	-	-	<0.2	-	-	-	-	-	-	-	-	-	-	-
Cole Slaw	91	122	1	13	8	7	-	-	-	-	-	-	-	-	-	-	-	-	-	-	-	-	-	-
Rolls	21	61	2	11	1	1	<5	0.10	0.04	1.0	-	-	0.3	-	-	-	-	-	-	-	-	-	-	-
Corn (5.5-inch ear)	135	169	5	31	3	X	162	0.12	0.07	1.2	-	-	2.6	-	-	-	-	-	-	-	-	-	-	-

* Includes two pieces of chicken, mashed potato and gravy, cole slaw, and roll. Source: Kentucky Fried Chicken, Inc. Louisville, Kentucky. Nutritional analysis by Raltech Scientific Services, Inc. (formerly WARF), Madison, Wisconsin.

Nutritional Analyses of Fast Foods

(Dashes indicate no data available. X = Less than 2% US RDA; tr=trace.)

	Wt (g)	Energy (kcal)	PRO (g)	CHO (g)	Fat (g)	Chol (mg)	A (IU)	B₁ (mg)	B₂ (mg)	Nia. (mg)	B₆ (mg)	B₁₂ (µg)	C (mg)	D (IU)	Ca (mg)	Cu (mg)	Fe (mg)	K (mg)	Mg (mg)	P (mg)	Na (mg)	Zn (mg)	Moisture (g)	Crude Fiber (g)
LONG JOHN SILVER'S®																								
Fish w/Batter (2 pc)	136	366	22	21	22	–	–	–	–	–	–	–	–	–	–	–	–	–	–	–	–	–	–	–
Fish w/Batter (3 pc)	207	549	32	32	32	–	–	–	–	–	–	–	–	–	–	–	–	–	–	–	–	–	–	–
Treasure Chest®	143	506	30	32	33	–	–	–	–	–	–	–	–	–	–	–	–	–	–	–	–	–	–	–
Chicken Planks® (4 pc)	166	457	27	35	23	–	–	–	–	–	–	–	–	–	–	–	–	–	–	–	–	–	–	–
Peg Legs® w/Batter (5 pc)	125	350	22	26	28	–	–	–	–	–	–	–	–	–	–	–	–	–	–	–	–	–	–	–
Ocean Scallops (6 pc)	120	283	11	30	13	–	–	–	–	–	–	–	–	–	–	–	–	–	–	–	–	–	–	–
Shrimp w/Batter (6 pc)	88	268	8	30	13	–	–	–	–	–	–	–	–	–	–	–	–	–	–	–	–	–	–	–
Breaded Oysters (6 pc)	156	441	13	53	19	–	–	–	–	–	–	–	–	–	–	–	–	–	–	–	–	–	–	–
Breaded Clams	142	617	18	61	34	–	–	–	–	–	–	–	–	–	–	–	–	–	–	–	–	–	–	–
Fish Sandwich	193	337	22	49	31	–	–	–	–	–	–	–	–	–	–	–	–	–	–	–	–	–	–	–
French Fryes	85	288	4	33	16	–	–	–	–	–	–	–	–	–	–	–	–	–	–	–	–	–	–	–
Cole Slaw	113	138	1	16	8	–	–	–	–	–	–	–	–	–	–	–	–	–	–	–	–	–	–	–
Corn on the Cob (1 ear)	150	176	5	29	4	–	–	–	–	–	–	–	–	–	–	–	–	–	–	–	–	–	–	–
Hushpuppies (3)	45	153	3	20	7	–	–	–	–	–	–	–	–	–	–	–	–	–	–	–	–	–	–	–
Clam Chowder (8 oz)	170	107	5	15	3	–	–	–	–	–	–	–	–	–	–	–	–	–	–	–	–	–	–	–

Source: Long John Silver's Food Shoppes, Lexington, Kentucky. Nutritional analysis by L. V. Packett, PhD. The Department of Nutrition and Food Science, University of Kentucky.

	Wt (g)	Energy (kcal)	PRO (g)	CHO (g)	Fat (g)	Chol (mg)	A (IU)	B₁ (mg)	B₂ (mg)	Nia. (mg)	B₆ (mg)	B₁₂ (µg)	C (mg)	D (IU)	Ca (mg)	Cu (mg)	Fe (mg)	K (mg)	Mg (mg)	P (mg)	Na (mg)	Zn (mg)	Moisture (g)	Crude Fiber (g)
McDONALD'S®																								
Egg McMuffin®	138	327	19	31	15	229	97	0.47	0.44	3.8	0.21	0.75	<1.4	46	226	0.12	2.9	168	26	322	885	1.9	70.7	0.1
English Muffin, Buttered	63	186	5	30	5	13	164	0.28	0.49	2.6	0.04	0.02	0.8	14	117	0.69	1.5	71	13	74	318	0.5	21.7	0.1
Hotcakes w/Butter & Syrup	214	500	8	94	10	47	257	0.26	0.36	2.3	0.12	0.19	4.7	31	103	0.11	2.2	187	28	501	1070	0.7	97.8	0.2
Sausage (Pork)	53	206	9	tr	19	43	<32	0.27	0.11	2.1	0.18	0.53	0.5	5	16	0.05	0.8	127	9	264	615	1.5	22.9	0.1
Scrambled Eggs	98	180	13	3	13	349	652	0.08	0.47	0.2	0.19	0.93	1.2	65	61	0.06	2.5	135	13	314	205	1.7	68.1	<0.1
Hashbrown Potatoes	55	125	2	14	7	7	<14	0.06	<0.01	0.8	0.13	0.01	4.1	<1	5	0.04	0.4	247	13	67	325	0.2	30.9	0.1
Big Mac®	204	563	26	41	33	86	530	0.39	0.37	6.5	0.27	1.8	2.2	33	157	0.18	4.0	237	38	314	1010	4.7	100.4	0.3
Cheeseburger	115	307	15	30	14	37	345	0.25	0.23	3.8	0.12	0.91	1.6	13	132	0.11	2.4	156	23	205	767	2.6	108.4	0.2
Hamburger	102	255	12	30	10	25	82	0.25	0.18	4.0	0.12	0.81	1.7	13	51	0.10	2.3	142	19	126	520	2.1	48.0	0.3
Quarter Pounder®	166	424	24	33	22	67	133	0.32	0.37	6.5	0.27	1.88	1.7	23	63	0.17	4.1	322	37	249	735	5.1	83.7	0.7
Quarter Pounder® w/Ch	194	524	30	32	31	96	660	0.31	0.37	7.4	0.23	2.15	2.7	25	219	0.18	4.3	341	41	382	1236	5.7	96.0	0.8
Filet-O-Fish®	139	432	14	37	25	47	42	0.26	0.20	2.6	0.10	0.82	<1.4	25	93	0.10	1.7	150	27	229	781	0.9	59.5	0.1
Regular Fries	68	220	3	26	12	9	<17	0.12	0.02	2.3	0.22	<0.03	12.5	<1	9	0.03	0.6	564	27	101	109	0.3	25.4	0.5
Apple Pie	85	253	2	29	14	12	<34	0.02	0.02	0.2	0.02	<0.04	<0.8	2	14	0.05	0.6	39	6	27	398	0.2	38.3	0.3
Cherry Pie	88	260	2	32	14	13	114	0.03	0.02	0.4	0.02	<0.02	<0.8	12	12	0.06	0.6	35	11	27	427	0.2	38.9	0.3
McDonaldland® Cookies	67	308	4	49	11	10	<27	0.23	0.23	2.9	0.03	0.03	0.9	10	12	0.07	1.5	52	11	74	358	0.3	2.2	0.1
Chocolate Shake	291	383	10	66	9	30	349	0.12	0.44	0.5	0.13	1.16	<2.9	44	320	0.19	0.8	580	49	335	300	1.4	203.0	0.3
Strawberry Shake	290	362	9	62	9	32	377	0.12	0.44	0.4	0.14	1.16	4.1	32	322	0.07	0.2	423	31	313	207	1.2	207.9	<0.3
Vanilla Shake	291	352	9	60	8	31	349	0.12	0.70	0.3	0.12	1.19	3.2	26	<329	0.09	0.6	410	31	314	201	1.2	211.3	0.3
Hot Fudge Sundae	164	310	7	46	11	18	230	0.07	0.31	1.1	0.13	0.7	2.5	16	215	0.13	0.2	236	35	236	175	1.0	97.9	0.2
Caramel Sundae	165	328	7	53	9	26	279	0.07	0.31	1.0	0.05	0.6	3.6	14	200	0.09	0.2	230	30	230	195	0.9	93.2	<0.2
Strawberry Sundae	164	289	7	46	9	20	230	0.07	0.30	1.0	0.05	0.6	2.8	16	174	0.11	0.4	290	28	80	96	0.8	101.0	0.2

Source: McDonald's Corporation, Oak Brook, Illinois. Nutritional analysis by Raltech Scientific Services, Inc. (formerly WARF), Madison, Wisconsin

TACO BELL*

Item																			
Bean Burrito	166	343	11	48	12	—	1657	0.37	0.22	2.2	—	15.2	98	2.8	235	173	272	—	—
Beef Burrito	184	466	30	37	21	—	1675	0.30	0.39	7.0	—	15.2	83	4.6	320	288	327	—	—
Beefy Tostada	184	291	19	21	15	—	3450	0.16	0.27	3.3	—	12.7	208	3.4	277	265	138	—	—
Bellbeefer*	123	221	19	23	7	—	2961	0.15	0.20	3.7	—	10.0	40	2.6	183	140	231	—	—
Bellbeefer* w/Ch	137	278	19	23	12	—	3146	0.16	0.27	3.7	—	10.0	147	2.7	195	208	330	—	—
Burrito Supreme*	225	457	21	43	22	—	3462	0.33	0.35	4.7	—	16.0	121	3.8	350	245	367	—	—
Combination Burrito	175	404	21	43	16	—	1666	0.34	0.31	4.6	—	15.2	91	3.7	278	230	300	—	—
Enchirito*	207	454	25	42	21	—	1178	0.31	0.37	4.7	—	9.5	259	3.8	491	338	1175	—	—
Pintos 'N Cheese	158	168	11	21	5	—	3123	0.26	0.16	0.9	—	9.3	150	2.3	307	210	102	—	—
Taco	83	186	15	14	8	—	120	0.09	0.16	2.9	—	0.2	120	2.5	143	175	79	—	—
Tostada	138	179	9	25	6	—	3152	0.18	0.15	0.8	—	9.7	191	2.3	172	186	101	—	—

Sources: 1) Menu Item Portions. San Antonio, Texas: Taco Bell Co. July 1976. 2) Adams CF. Nutritive value of American foods in common units, in Handbook No. 456. Washington USDA Agricultural Research Service November 1975. 3) Church EF, Church HN (eds). Food Values of Portions Commonly Used, ed 12. Philadelphia. JB Lippincott Co. 1975. 4) Valley Baptist Medical Center Food Service Department. Descriptions of Mexican-American Foods. Fort Atkinson, Wisconsin. NASCO.

WENDY'S*

Item																			
Single Hamburger	200	470	26	34	26	70	94	0.24	0.36	5.8	0.6		84	5.3	239	774	4.8	110.6	0.8
Double Hamburger	285	670	44	34	40	125	128	0.43	0.54	10.6	1.5		138	8.2	364	980	8.4	162.1	1.1
Triple Hamburger	360	850	65	33	51	205	220	0.47	0.68	14.7	2.0		104	10.7	525	1217	13.5	204.6	1.4
Single w/Cheese	240	580	33	34	34	90	221	0.38	0.43	6.3	0.7		228	5.4	315	1085	5.5	133.4	1.0
Double w/Cheese	325	800	50	41	48	155	439	0.49	0.75	11.4	2.3		177	10.2	489	1414	10.1	179.2	1.3
Triple w/Cheese	400	1040	72	35	68	225	472	0.80	0.84	15.1	3.4		371	10.9	712	1848	14.3	216.4	1.6
Chili	250	230	19	21	8	25	1188	0.22	0.25	3.4	2.9		83	4.4	168	1065	3.7	195.9	1.6
French Fries	120	330	5	41	16	5	40	0.14	0.07	X	6.4		16	1.2	196	112	0.5	54.9	2.3
Frosty	250	390	9	54	16	45	355	0.20	0.60	3.0	0.7	X	270	0.9	278	247	1.0	169.8	0.0

Source: Wendy's International, Inc. Dublin, Ohio. Nutritional analysis by Medallion Laboratories, Minneapolis, Minnesota.

PIZZA

Item																			
Pizza, cheese 1 slice	100	239	13	28	8	—	141	0.16	0.24	1.7	—		225	1.3	233	33	215	585	—
Pizza, thick crust, 10 inch	417	919	46	156	12	—	—	—	—	—	—		579	5.2	947	156	637	2265	—
Cheese pizza, thin crust 10 inch	336	718	37	98	19	—	560	0.09	0.12	1.5	—	9	710	2.2	570	79	669	2232	—
Pepperoni pizza 1 slice	100	234	8	29	9	—	—	—	—	—	—		17	1.2	168	92	—	729	—

Nutritional Analyses of Fast Foods

(Dashes indicate no data available. X = Less than 2% US RDA; tr=trace.)

	Wt (g)	Energy (kcal)	PRO (g)	CHO (g)	Fat (g)	Chol (mg)	Vitamins								Minerals								Caffeine (mg)	Sac-char. (mg)
							A (IU)	B₁ (mg)	B₂ (mg)	Nia. (mg)	B₆ (mg)	B₁₂ (µg)	C (mg)	D (IU)	Ca (mg)	Cu (mg)	Fe (mg)	K (mg)	Mg (mg)	P (mg)	Na (mg)	Zn (mg)		
BEVERAGES																								
Coffee*	180	2	tr	tr	tr	–	0	0	tr	0.5	–	–	0	–	4	–	0.2	65	–	7	2	–	100†	0
Tea*	180	2	tr	tr	tr	–	0	0	0.04	0.1	–	–	1	–	5	–	0.2	–	18	4	–	–	40†	0
Orange Juice	183	82	1	20	tr	–	366	0.17	0.02	0.6	–	–	82.4	–	17	–	0.2	340	–	29	2	–	–	0
Chocolate Milk	250	213	9	28	9	–	330	0.08	0.40	0.3	–	–	3.0	–	278	–	0.5	365	–	235	118	–	–	0
Skim Milk	245	88	9	13	tr	–	10	0.09	0.44	0.2	–	–	2.0	–	296	–	0.1	355	–	233	127	–	–	0
Whole Milk	244	159	9	12	9	27	342	0.07	0.41	0.2	–	–	2.4	100	188	–	tr	351	32	227	122	–	28	0
Coca-Cola®	246	96	0	24	0	0	–	–	–	–	–	–	–	–	–	–	–	–	–	40	20‡	–	28	0
Fanta® Ginger Ale	244	84	0	21	0	0	–	–	–	–	–	–	–	–	–	–	–	–	–	–	30‡	–	0	0
Fanta® Grape	247	114	0	29	0	0	–	–	–	–	–	–	–	–	–	–	–	–	–	–	21‡	–	0	0
Fanta® Orange	248	117	0	30	0	0	–	–	–	–	–	–	–	–	–	–	–	–	–	–	21‡	–	0	0
Fanta® Root Beer	246	103	0	27	0	0	–	–	–	–	–	–	–	–	–	–	–	–	–	–	23‡	–	0	0
Mr. Pibb®	245	95	0	25	0	0	–	–	–	–	–	–	–	–	–	–	–	–	–	29	23‡	–	27	0
Mr. Pibb® w/o Sugar	236	1	0	tr	0	0	–	–	–	–	–	–	–	–	–	–	–	–	–	28	37‡	–	38	76
Sprite®	245	95	0	24	0	0	–	–	–	–	–	–	–	–	–	–	–	–	–	–	42‡	–	0	0
Sprite® w/o Sugar	236	3	0	0	0	0	–	–	–	–	–	–	–	–	–	–	–	–	–	–	42‡	–	0	57
Tab®	236	tr	0	tr	0	0	–	–	–	–	–	–	–	–	–	–	–	–	–	30	30‡	–	30	74
Fresca®	236	tr	0	0	0	–	–	–	–	–	–	–	–	–	–	–	–	–	–	–	38‡	–	0	54

*6-oz serving; all other data are for 8-oz serving. †Caffeine content depends on strength of beverage. ‡Value when bottling water with average sodium content (12 mg/8 oz) is used. Sources: 1) Adams CF Nutritive value of American foods in common units, in *Handbook* No. 456. Washington. USDA Agricultural Research Service. November 1975; 2) The Coca-Cola Company. Atlanta. Georgia. January 1977; 3) *American Hospital Formulary Service*. Washington. American Society of Hospital Pharmacists. Section 28:20. March 1978.

APPENDIX

Ⓑ

Natural Toxins in Food

Everybody is talking about eating unprocessed and whole foods. There is concern about the harmful effects of additives and we are mindful of the dangers of environmental pollutants. But have you ever thought that carrots, peanuts, whole-grain cereals, or potatoes could endanger your health? All of these contain naturally occurring *toxicants*—substances that occur naturally and that can cause adverse reactions if eaten in unusually large amounts.

Natural toxicants in food are unfamiliar to most of us but they have been important sources of human illness and death throughout history. Potato poisoning was common in areas of the world where potatoes were eaten in large amounts in times of food shortages. African populations who eat large amounts of bananas have a high incidence of heart lesions. And a few cases of mushroom poisoning are reported yearly to the National Clearinghouse for Poison Control. Are we suggesting no more potatoes, bananas, or mushrooms? Not at all.

We are discussing toxicants as one more example of a risk factor. Health lies not in avoiding all risks but in minimizing them.

All foods listed below are safe when eaten as part of a balanced and varied diet. Their potential risk is tiny but none the less present. Overenthusiastic or unskilled imitators of naturalists, food faddists, or those who eat bizarre diets may face greater jeopardy. Most of us do not.

Substance	Food Source	Toxic Effect	Comments
Goitrogens	cabbage, kale, Brussels sprouts, cauliflower, broccoli, turnips, watercress, radish	induce goiter by interfering with the body's use of iodine	Cooking these vegetables inactivates goitrogenic activity.

303

Substance	Food Source	Toxic Effect	Comments
Estrogens	soybeans, soybean sprouts, alfalfa, carrots, wheat, rice, oats, barley, potatoes, apples, cherries, cottonseed oil, safflower oil, wheat germ oil, olive oil	responsible for cases of livestock infertility	Quantity of estrogen present is too low to cause any effect in the body.
Vasoactive amines tyramine dopamine norepinephrine serotonin histamine	plantains, bananas, ripened cheese, avocados, soybeans, meat broth, liver, pineapple juice	elevation in blood pressure; migraine headaches	These amines are usually inactivated by an enzyme normally present in body; mood-elevating drugs can inhibit this enzyme.
Trypsin inhibitor	soybeans, lima beans, mung beans, peanuts, oats, buckwheat, barley, sweet potato, peas, corn, white potato	interferes with digestion and absorption of protein	Cooking destroys the inhibitor.
Solanin	potatoes (most potent), apples, eggplant	interferes with transmission of nerve impulses; poisoning	Not destroyed in cooking— found mainly in skins.
Alkaoloidlike compounds and cyclopeptides	mushrooms	poisoning	Only a small number of mushroom species are poisonous; domestically cultivated mushrooms are free of toxic substances; never harvest mushrooms from an unknown source.

Substance	Food Source	Toxic Effect	Comments
Cyanide	apricot pits or kernels, peach pits, kernel paste, cassava, cashew nuts, lima beans, kirsch liqueur	cyanide poisoning	The controversial cancer treatment Laetrile is made with apricot kernels.
Glycyrrhizic acid	licorice	severe hypertension, water retention, enlarged heart	Daily eating of large amounts of licorice candy has caused some symptoms; not found in artificially flavored licorice.
Menthol	candy, gums, liqueurs, cigarettes, toothpaste, mouthwash	hives, heart fibrillation, psychosis	Severe symptoms have been reported due to addiction to mentholated cigarettes or peppermint candy.
Myristicin	nutmeg, mace, black pepper, carrots, parsley, celery, dill	headache, cramps, nausea, poisoning	Large amounts of nutmeg or mace result in symptoms similar to drunkenness and can be poisonous.
Aflatoxins	peanuts, peanut butter, other nuts, corn, wheat	liver damage; carcinogenic	Domestic peanuts and imported nuts are monitored for contamination.
Antivitamins avidin	egg whites	Inactivates biotin	An antivitamin diminishes or destroys the effect of a vitamin in the body; avidin and some forms of thiaminase are destroyed by cooking.

Substance	Food Source	Toxic Effect	Comments
thiaminase	blackberries, black currants, red beets, Brussels sprouts, red cabbage, spinach, raw fish	inactivates thiamine (B_1)	
citral	orange peel, marmalade	inhibits vitamin A	
Safrole	oil of sassafras	carcinogenic	Prohibited in our food supply since 1958.
Thujone	herbal teas containing sage, yarrow or wormwood, vermouth	poisoning, convulsions	Allergic reactions have occurred from chronic use of herbal teas with yarrow.
Psoralens	parsley, parsnips, figs, limes, caraway	photosensitizers resulting in unusual sensitivity to sun causing severe sunburn	Large portion destroyed in cooking.
Benzopyrene	charcoal-broiled meat, olive oil, smoked meats	carcinogenic	See Chapter 9 for more information
Nitrates	beets, spinach, radishes, lettuce, drinking water	carcinogenic	See Chapter 9 for more information.
Phenols	rhubarb, St. John's-wort, buckwheat, cashew, mangos, nutmeg, sassafras, honey, apples	poisoning	Plant poisonings are responsible for 4% of all accidental poisonings each year— most occur in small children

Substance	Food Source	Toxic Effect	Comments
Oxalates	spinach, swiss chard, beets, greens, rhubarb	inhibits absorption of calcium	Rhubarb leaves contain 3 to 4 times as much as stalk and can result in illness if eaten raw.
Phytate	cereals, nuts, dried peas and beans, wheat germ	inhibits absorption of calcium, zinc, iron, magnesium	High-fiber diets are rich in phytates.

Diabetic Exchange Lists for Meal Planning

One of the most important aspects of diabetes management is dietary care. The Food Exchanges are lists of foods grouped by similar values of carbohydrates, proteins, and fats so that they can be substituted in your daily meal plans. Foods have been divided into six categories: milks, vegetables, fruits, breads, meats, and fats. Foods in any one group can be substituted or exchanged with other foods within the same group.

BREAD EXCHANGES: One Exchange of Bread contains 15 gm of carbohydrate, 2 gm of protein, and 70 calories.

Bread

White (including French and Italian)	1 slice
Whole Wheat	1 slice
Rye or Pumpernickel	1 slice
Raisin	1 slice
Bagel, small	½
English Muffin, small	½
Plain Roll, bread	1
Frankfurter Roll	½
Hamburger Bun	½
Dried Bread Crumbs	3 Tbs
Tortilla, 6″	1

Cereal

Bran Flakes	½ cup
Other ready-to-eat unsweetened cereal	¾ cup
Puffed Cereal (unfrosted)	1 cup
Cereal (cooked)	½ cup
Grits (cooked)	½ cup
Rice or Barley (cooked)	½ cup
Pasta (cooked), Noodles, Spaghetti, Macaroni	½ cup
Popcorn (popped, no fat added	3 cups
Cornmeal (dry)	2 Tbs
Flour	2½ Tbs
Wheat Germ	¼ cup

Crackers		Prepared Foods	
Arrowroot	3	Biscuit, 2" dia.	1
Graham, 2½" sq.	2	(omit 1 Fat Exchange)	
Matzoh, 4" × 6"	½ cup	Corn Bread, 2" × 2" × 1"	1
Oyster	20	(omit 1 Fat Exchange)	
Pretzels, 3-1/8" long	25	Corn Muffin, 2" dia.	1
× 1/8" dia.		(omit 1 Fat Exchange)	
Rye Wafers, 2" × 3½"	3	Crackers, round butter type	5
Saltines	6	(omit 1 Fat Exchange)	
Soda, 2½" sq.	4	Muffin, plain small	1
		(omit 1 Fat Exchange)	
Dried Beans, Peas, and		Potatoes, French Fried,	8
Lentils		length 2" to 3½"	
Beans, Peas, Lentils	½ cup	(omit 1 Fat Exchange)	
(dried and cooked)		Potato or Corn Chips	15
Baked Beans, no pork	¼ cup	(omit 2 Fat Exchanges)	
(canned)		Pancake, 5" × ½"	1
		(omit 1 Fat Exchange)	
Starchy Vegetables		Waffle, 5" × ½"	1
Corn	⅓ cup	(omit 1 Fat Exchange)	

VEGETABLE EXCHANGES: One Exchange of Vegetables contains about 5 gm of carbohydrate, 2 gm of protein, and 25 calories. One Exchange is ½ cup.

Asparagus	Greens:	Rhubarb
Bean Sprouts	Beet	Rutabaga
Beets	Chards	Sauerkraut
Broccoli	Collards	String Beans
Brussels Sprouts	Dandelion	(green or yellow)
Cabbage	Kale	Summer Squash
Carrots	Mustard	Tomatoes
Cauliflower	Spinach	Tomato Juice
Celery	Turnip	Turnips
Cucumbers	Mushrooms	Vegetable Juice Cocktail
Eggplant	Okra	Zucchini
Green Pepper	Onions	

The following raw vegetables may be used as desired:

Chicory	Lettuce
Chinese Cabbage	Parsley
Endive	Radishes
Escarole	Watercress

Starchy Vegetables are found in the Bread Exchange List

FRUIT EXCHANGES: One Exchange of Fruit contains 10 gm of carbohydrate and 40 calories.

Apple	1 small	Mango	½ small
Apple Juice	⅓ cup	Melon	
Applesauce (unsweetened)	½ cup	Cantaloupe	¼ small
Apricots, fresh	2 med.	Honeydew	⅛ med.
Apricots, dried	4 halves	Watermelon	1 cup
Banana	½ small	Nectarine	1 small
Berries		Orange	1 small
Blackberries	½ cup	Orange Juice	½ cup
Blueberries	½ cup	Papaya	¾ cup
Raspberries	½ cup	Peach	1 med.
Strawberries	¾ cup	Pear	1 small
Cherries	10 large	Persimmon, native	1 med.
Cider	⅓ cup	Pineapple	½ cup
Dates	2	Pineapple Juice	⅓ cup
Figs, fresh	1	Plums	2 med.
Figs, dried	1	Prunes	2 med.
Grapefruit	½	Prune Juice	¼ cup
Grapefruit Juice	½ cup	Raisins	2 Tbs
Grapes	12	Tangerine	1 med.
Grape Juice	¼ cup		

Cranberries may be used as desired if no sugar is added.

MEAT EXCHANGES:

LEAN MEAT: One Exchange of Lean Meat (1 oz) contains 7 gm of protein, 3 gm of fat, and 55 calories.

Beef:	Baby Beef (very lean), Chipped Beef, Chuck, Flank Steak, Tenderloin, Plate Ribs, Plate Skirt Steak, Round (bottom top), All cuts Rump, Spare Ribs, Tripe	1 oz
Lamb:	Leg, Rib, Sirloin, Loin (roast and chops), Shank, Shoulder	1 oz
Pork:	Leg (Whole Rump, Center Shank), Ham Smoked (center slices)	1 oz
Veal:	Leg, Loin, Rib, Shank, Shoulder, Cutlets	1 oz
Poultry:	Meat without skin of Chicken, Turkey, Cornish Hen, Guinea Hen, Pheasant	1 oz
Fish:	Any fresh or frozen	1 oz
	Canned Salmon, Tuna, Mackerel, Crab, and Lobster	¼ cup
	Clams, Oysters, Scallops, Shrimp	5, or 1 oz
	Sardines, drained	3

Cheeses containing less than 5 percent butterfat		1 oz
Cottage cheese, dry and 2 percent butterfat		¼ cup
Dried Beans and Peas (omit 1 Bread Exchange)		½ cup

MEDIUM-FAT MEAT: For each Exchange of Medium-Fat Meat omit ½ Fat Exchange.

Beef:	Ground (15 percent fat), Corned Beef (canned), Rib Eye, Round (ground commercial)	1 oz
Pork:	Loin (all cuts Tenderloin), Shoulder Arm (picnic) Shoulder Blade, Boston Butt, Canadian Bacon, Boiled Ham	1 oz
Liver, Heart, Kidney and Sweetbreads (these are high in cholesterol)		1 oz
Cottage cheese, creamed		¼ cup
Cheese: Mozzarella, Ricotta, Farmer's Cheese, Neufchatel, Parmesan		3 Tbs
Egg (high in cholesterol)		1
Peanut Butter (omit 2 additional Fat Exchanges)		2 Tbs

HIGH-FAT MEAT: For each Exchange of High-Fat Meat omit 1 Fat Exchange.

Beef:	Brisket, Corned Beef (Brisket), Ground Beef (more than 20 percent fat), Hamburger (commercial), Chuck (ground commercial), Roasts (Rib), Steaks (Club and Rib)	1 oz
Lamb:	Breast	1 oz
Pork:	Spare Ribs, Loin (Back Ribs), Pork (ground), Country-style Ham, Deviled Ham	1 oz
Veal:	Breast	1 oz
Poultry:	Capon, Duck (domestic), Goose	1 oz
Cheese:	Cheddar Types	1 oz
Cold Cuts		4½″ × ⅛″ slice
Frankfurter		1 small

MILK EXCHANGES: One Exchange of Milk contains 12 gm of carbohydrate, 8 gm of protein, a trace of fat, and 80 calories.

NON-FAT FORTIFIED MILK

Skim or nonfat milk	1 cup
Powdered (nonfat dry, before adding liquid)	⅓ cup
Canned, evaporated skim milk	½ cup
Buttermilk made from skim milk	1 cup
Yogurt made from skim milk (plain, unflavored)	1 cup

LOW-FAT FORTIFIED MILK

1 percent fat fortified milk (omit ½ Fat Exchange)	1 cup
2 percent fat fortified milk (omit 1 Fat Exchange)	1 cup
Yogurt made from 2 percent fortified milk (plain, unflavored) (omit 1 Fat Exchange)	1 cup

WHOLE MILK (omit 2 Fat Exchanges)

Whole milk	1 cup
Canned, evaporated whole milk	½ cup
Buttermilk made from whole milk	1 cup
Yogurt made from whole milk (plain, unflavored)	1 cup

FAT EXCHANGES: One Exchange of Fat contains 5 gm of fat and 45 calories.

POLYUNSATURATED		SATURATED	
Margarine, soft, tub or stick*	1 Tsp	Margarine, regular stick	1 Tsp
Avocado (4″ dia.)**	1/8	Butter	1 Tsp
Oil, Corn, Cottonseed, Safflower, Soy, Sunflower	1 Tsp	Bacon fat	1 Tsp
		Bacon crisp	1 strip
Oil, Olive**	1 Tsp	Cream, light	2 Tbs
Oil, Peanut**	1 Tsp	Cream, sour	2 Tbs
Olives**	5 small	Cream, heavy	1 Tbs
Almonds**	10 whole	Cream cheese	1 Tbs
Pecans**	2 large whole	French dressing***	1 Tbs
Peanuts, Spanish**	20 whole	Italian dressing***	1 Tbs
Peanuts, Virginia**	10 whole	Lard	1 Tsp
Walnuts	6 small	Mayonnaise***	1 Tsp
Nuts, other**	6 small	Salad dressing, Mayonnaise-type***	2 Tsp
		Salt Pork	¾″ cube

*Made with corn, cottonseed, safflower, soy or sunflower oil only.

**Fat content is primarily monounsaturated.

***If made with corn, cottonseed, safflower, soy or sunflower oil can be used on fat-modified diet.

GENERAL RULES

FREE FOODS

Seasonings: Cinnamon, celery salt, garlic, garlic salt, lemon, mustard, ming, nutmeg, parsley, pepper, sugarless sweeteners, spices, vanilla, and vinegar.

Other foods: Coffee or tea (without sugar or cream), fat-free broth, bouillon, unflavored gelatin, sour or dill pickles, cranberries (without sugar).

FOODS TO AVOID

Sugar, candy, honey, jam, jelly, marmalade, syrups, pie, cake, cookies, pastries, condensed milk, soft drinks, candy-coated gum; fried, scalloped or creamed foods; beer, wine, or other alcoholic beverages.

Source: The Exchange Lists are based on material in the *Exchange Lists for Planning,* prepared by the Committees of the American Diabetes Association, Inc., and the American Dietetic Association in cooperation with the National Institute of Arthritis, Metabolism, and Digestive Diseases and the National Heart and Lung Institute, National Institutes of Health, Public Health Service, U.S. Department of Health, Education and Welfare.

Fast Food Exchanges for Diabetics and Dieters

Many of us eat in fast food restaurants often. Every week 52 percent of all the fast food meals are eaten by people over forty. We spend over $7 billion a year on these standardized food items. This list of nutritional values and numbers of exchanges in popular food selections will guide you, whether diabetic or not, so you can intelligently choose foods that will fit in with the other meals you eat. Fast foods can be part of a well-rounded, nutritious diet.

	NUTRITIONAL VALUES				EXCHANGES		
	CAL.	CARB (Grams)	PRO. (Grams)	FAT (Grams)	BREAD	MEAT (Medium)	FAT*
ARTHUR TREACHER'S							
(fish, chips, coleslaw)							
3-piece dinner	1100	91	38	65	6	4	9
2-piece dinner	905	83	28	51	5½	2½	8
BURGER CHEF							
Hamburger	250	23	12	12	1½	1	1½
Cheeseburger	304	24	14	17	1½	1½	2
Double Hamburger	325	28	20	15	2	2½	½
Double Cheeseburger	434	24	24	26	1½	3	2
Big Shef	535	41	25	30	2¾	3	3
Super Shef	600	39	29	37	2½	3½	4
Skipper's Treat	604	39	29	37	2½	3	4½
Rancher Platter	640	44	30	38	3	3½	4
Mariner Platter	680	85	32	24	5½	3	2
French fries	187	25	3	9	1½	—	2
Milkshake, Chocolate	310	48	9	9	3	½	1
BURGER KING							
Hamburger	310	30	16	14	2	1½	1½
Hamburger with cheese	360	31	19	18	2	2	1½
Double meat hamburger	440	32	26	23	2	3	1½
Double meat hamburger with cheese	540	33	31	32	2	4	2½
Whopper	650	51	27	37	3½	3	4½
Double Beef Whopper	850	54	44	52	3½	5	5½
Whopper with cheese	760	54	33	46	3½	3½	5½
Double Beef Whopper with cheese	970	55	50	61	3½	6	6
Whopper Jr.	360	31	15	20	2	1½	2½
Whopper Jr. with cheese	420	32	18	24	2	2	3
Whopper Jr. with double meat	490	32	25	29	2	3	3
Whopper Jr. double meat pattie with cheese	550	33	28	34	2	3½	3½
Whaler	660	54	28	37	3½	3	4½
Whaler with cheese	770	55	33	46	3½	3½	5½
Steak Sandwich	600	64	39	21	4	4½	—
Onion Rings	230	24	3	13	1½	—	2½
French Fries	240	28	3	12	2	—	2½
Milk Shake, Choc.	380	62	9	11	4	—	2
Milk Shake, Vanilla	360	55	9	11	3½	½	2

* At first glance, some fat exchanges may seem too low. Look at the meat calculation, the fat content may be included there.

		NUTRITIONAL VALUES			EXCHANGES		
	CAL.	CARB. (Grams)	PRO. (Grams)	FAT (Grams)	BREAD	MEAT (Medium)	FAT
KENTUCKY FRIED CHICKEN							
(fried chicken, mashed potato, coleslaw, rolls)							
3-piece dinner							
Original	830	61	50	43	4	6	2½
Crispy	1070	74	54	62	5	6½	6
2-piece dinner							
Original	595	51	35	28	3½	4	1½
Crispy	665	40	37	40	2½	4½	3½
LONG JOHN SILVER							
(fish, chips, coleslaw)							
3-piece dinner	1190	100	55	63	7	6	7
2-piece dinner	955	89	38	50	6	3½	6
McDONALD'S							
Hamburger	260	31	14	9	1½	1	1½
Cheeseburger	306	31	16	13	2	2	1
Quarter Pounder	418	33	26	21	2	3	1
Quarter Pounder with cheese	518	34	31	29	2½	3½	2
Big Mac	550	44	21	32	3	2	4
Filet-O-Fish	402	34	15	23	2½	1½	3
French fries	211	26	3	11	2	—	2
Egg McMuffin	352	26	18	20	2	2	2
Pork Sausage	184	trace	9	17	—	1	2½
Scrambled Eggs	162	2	12	12	—	1½	1
Shake, Chocolate	364	60	11	9	4	½	1
PIZZA HUT							
(cheese pizza)							
individual							
thick crust	1030	143	71	19	9½	6	—
thin crust	1005	128	61	28	8½	6	—
½ of 13-inch							
thick crust	900	113	65	21	7½	6	—
thin crust	850	103	50	26	7	5	—
1 slice (⅛ of pie)	225	26	12½	6½	2	2	—
½ of 15-inch							
thick crust	1200	148	83	31	10	7	—
thin crust	1150	144	66	35	9½	7	—
SUBMARINE HERO GRINDER							
(8-inch sandwich)							
Italian cold cuts	620	60	36	26	4	4	1
Roast Beef	600	55	46	22	3½	5	—
Tuna	700	55	41	34	3½	5	2
TACO BELL							
Bean Burrito	343	48	11	12	3	1	2
Beef Burrito	466	37	30	21	2½	3½	½
Beefy Tostada	291	21	19	15	1½	2½	½
Bellbeefer	221	23	15	7	1½	2	—
Bellbeefer with cheese	278	23	19	12	1½	2	½
Burrito Supreme	457	43	21	22	3	2	2½
Combination Burrito	404	43	21	16	3	2	1
Enchirito	454	42	25	21	3	3	1½
Pintos 'n Cheese	168	21	11	5	1½	1	—
Taco	186	14	15	8	1	2	—
Tostada	179	25	9	6	2	1	—

SOURCE: Wendy Midgley, R. D. "Eat on the Fast Food Trail," *Diabetes Forecast,* July–August, 1979, p. 20.

Food Additives

Additives are not new. Ancient man preserved foods by smoking and salting or coating his food with spices. Hams were pierced with cloves so they could be kept longer. No one knew why this was done, but it worked. The reason that the clove-studded ham stored well was because cloves contain *eugenol*, a chemical that inhibits bacterial growth. The word EUGENOL on a food label would arouse suspicion, while cloves does not.

The first federal food safety laws were enacted in 1906 to stop wide-scale adulteration of foods. To test the safety of a food additive during this era, the Agricultural Department's Bureau of Chemistry employed a squad of food-testing volunteers who ate pure foods that were laced with such substances as borax, benzoic acid, and formaldehyde. Human testing today is impossible for ethical and practical reasons.

Scientists who evaluate new and reevaluate old additives use laboratory animals. Short-term tests determine toxicity. If a lethal dose is low, the additive probably will never be used for human consumption. Long-term tests that evaluate the effects of lifetime consumption take a minimum of two years to complete and must be done on at least two species of animals.

Animal testing is often criticized, especially when the animals are fed huge test doses of a substance. It is true that men and animals differ, but if a substance makes an animal sick or causes harm there is a good chance it will cause problems in humans as well. Even if results overemphasize dangers, because huge doses were fed and/or results from animals were applied to man, the error, if any, would be on the side of safety. This type of scientific bias helps to protect the consumer by establishing a wide margin of safety in the dose levels allowed for use when an additive is approved. Consequently, few new additives are approved.

In 1980 the government concluded an extensive reevaluation of additives currently in use. Four-hundred-fifteen substances were on the GRAS (Generally Recognized As Safe) list because they seemed, by virtue of long-term use, to be safe. After reevaluation, 305 items retained their safe status. Sixty-eight substances were classified safe at current levels of use but would require further study. Zinc salts, alginates, iron and iron salts, tannic acid, sucrose, and vitamins A and D were in this group. Nineteen substances are being more carefully controlled until unresolved questions are answered by further research. BHA and BHT are examples in this category. Twenty-five substances needed either new guidelines for use or required some research before any recommendations could be issued. Salt, some modified food starches, glycerides, and carnauba wax (used in cosmetics and drugs) are a few of these questionable substances. The FDA is currently implementing new regulations for GRAS ingredients to ensure the safe use of additives in our food supply.

Consumers, however, are still not convinced of the safety of additives. Public opinion polls show that over half favor elimination of additives—even if that results in less-appealing foods. Such alarm is probably not warranted. Since fear is often generated by the unknown, the following chart should help you to be a more informed consumer. It will help you understand why the additive is used and the products it is used in.

ADDITIVES IN FOODS

Preservatives—prevent unappetizing changes in color, flavor and texture when food is exposed to air; may block poisonous effect of microorganisms.

Additive	*Used in*	*Function*
Alpha-tocopherol	vegetable oil	antioxidant
Ascorbic acid erythorbic acid sodium ascorbate sodium erythorbate	oily food cereal soft drinks cured meat	antioxidant color stabilizer
BHA (butylated hydroxyanisole)	cereals chewing gum baking mixes snack chips instant potatoes	antioxidant

317

Additive	Used in	Function
BHT (butylated hydroxytoluene)	same as above	antioxidant
Calcium propionate or sodium propionate	bread rolls pie cakes	prevents mold growth
Citric acid sodium citrate	ice cream sherbet fruit drinks candy soft drinks instant potatoes gelatin desserts jam	antioxidant acidifier flavoring agent chelating agent
Lactic acid	Spanish olive cheese frozen desserts soft drinks	acidifier flavoring agent
Lecithin	baked goods margarine salad dressing chocolate ice cream	emulsifier antioxidant
Propyl gallate	vegetable oil meat products potato snacks chicken soup base chewing gum	antioxidant
Sodium hypophosphite	bacon frankfurters smoked meat ham	preservative
Sodium benzoate	fruit juice soft drinks pickles preserves	inhibits growth of microorganisms

318

Additive	Used in	Function
Sodium nitrate	ham frankfurters luncheon meat corned beef	coloring agent flavoring agent
Sodium nitrite	smoked fish bacon	preservative
Sorbic acid postassium sor- bate	cheese syrup jelly cakes wines dry fruit	prevents growth of mold and bacteria
Sulfur dioxide sodium bisulfite	sliced fruit wine grape juice dehydrated potatoes	prevents bacterial growth bleaching agent

Processing agents—aid in the production of food by improving taste or texture.

Additive	Used in	Function
Alginate propylene glycol alginate	ice cream cheese candy yogurt soft drinks salad dressing beer	thickening agent foam stabilizer
Calcium stearoyl lactylate Sodium stearoyl lactylate Sodium stearoyl fumarate	bread dough cake filling artificial whipped topping	dough conditioner whipping agent
Carrageenan	ice cream jelly chocolate milk infant formula	thickening agent stabilizing agent

Additive	Used in	Function
Casein sodium caseinate	sherbet ice cream candy soft drinks instant potatoes	whitening agent thickening agent
Dipotassium phos- phate	cold cereals	chelating agent

EDTA
   ethylenediamine
   tetraacetic acid
	salad dressing
	margarine
	sandwich spread
	mayonnaise
	processed fruits
	   and vegetables
	canned shellfish
	soft drinks
		chelating agent

Gelatin	powdered dessert mixes yogurt ice cream cheese spread beverages	thickening agent gelling agent

Glycerin
   glycerol
	marshmallows
	candy
	fudge
	baked goods
		maintains water
		   content

Gums
   guar
   locust bean
   arabic
   tragacanth
   acacia
	beverages
	ice cream
	frozen pudding
	salad dressing
	dough
	cottage cheese
	candy
	drink mixes
		thickening agents
		stabilizers

Modified food starch	soup gravy baby food	thickening agent

Additive	Used in	Function
Monoglycerides Diglycerides	baked goods margarine candy peanut butter	emulsifier
Pectin	jelly jam soft cheese	stabilizer thickener
Phosphoric acid phosphates	baked goods cheese powdered foods cured meat soda pop breakfast cereal dehydrated potatoes	acidulant chelating agent buffer emulsifier discoloration inhibitor
Polydextrose	frozen desserts cakes candies	bulking agent
Polysorbate 60	baked goods frozen desserts imitation dairy products	emulsifier
Sodium carboxymethyl cellulose methyl cellulose carboxymethyl cellulose (CMC)	ice cream beer pie filling icing diet food candy	thickening agent stabilizing agent prevents sugar from crystallizing
Sodium silicoaluminate	salt baking powder sugar	antifoaming agent anticaking agent
Sorbitan monostearate	cakes candy frozen pudding icing	emulsifier

Flavorings—Sugar and salt make up 140 of the 150 pounds of additives eaten annually. Both are natural flavorings. Other flavoring agents are eaten in far smaller amounts.

Additive	Used in	Function
Artificial flavoring	soda pop candy breakfast cereal gelatin desserts many processed foods	flavoring
Aspartame	cold breakfast cereal chewing gum drink mixes instant coffee and tea gelatin pudding pie filling nondairy whipped topping	noncaloric sweetener
Corn syrup corn syrup solids	candy toppings syrup snack food imitation dairy foods coffee whitener	sweetener thickener
Dextrose glucose corn sugar	bread caramel soft drinks cookies many processed foods	sweetener coloring agent
Fumaric acid	powdered drinks pudding pie filling gelatin desserts	tartness agent

Additive	Used in	Function
Hydrolyzed vegetable protein (HVP)	instant soups frankfurters sauce mixes beef stew	flavor enhancer
Invert sugar	candy soft drinks many processed foods	sweetener
Lactose	whipped topping mix breakfast pastry	sweetener
Mannitol	chewing gum low-calorie food	sweetener
Monosodium glutamate (MSG)	soup seafood poultry cheese sauces many processed foods	flavor enhancer
Quinine	tonic water quinine water bitter lemon	flavoring
Saccharin	diet food and drinks	noncaloric sweetener
Salt sodium chloride	most processed food	flavoring
Sorbitol	diet food and drinks candy shredded coconut chewing gum	sweetener thickening agent maintains moisture
Sugar sucrose	table sugar sweetened food	sweetener

Additive	Used in	Function
Vanillin ethyl vanillin	ice cream baked goods beverages chocolate candy gelatin desserts	substitute for vanilla

Colorings—colors for foods may be synthetic or natural.

Artificial Colors Red No. 3	cherries in fruit cocktail candy baked goods	coloring agent
Red No. 40	soft drinks candy gelatin desserts pastry pet food sausages	coloring agent
Blue No. 1	baked goods beverages candy	coloring agent
Blue No. 2	pet food beverages candy	coloring agent
Yellow No. 5 Egg shade	gelatin dessert candy pet food baked goods	coloring agent
Yellow No. 6	beverages sausage baked goods candy gelatin	coloring agent
Green No. 3	candy beverages	coloring agent

Additive	Used in	Function
Beet powder	cooked meats	coloring agent
tomato powder	cheese	
Beta carotene	margarine	coloring agent
carotene	butter	
	coffee whiteners	
Caramel	baked products	coloring agent
	ice cream	flavoring agent
	soft drinks	
	candy	
	meat	
	syrup	
	rum	
	brandy	
	root beer	
Chlorophyll	toothpaste	coloring agent
	mouthwash	
Ferrous gluconate	black olives	coloring agent
Riboflavin	coffee whiteners	coloring agent
		nutrient

Height-Weight Table

DESIRABLE WEIGHTS FOR MEN AGED 25 AND OVER
(WEIGHT IN POUNDS ACCORDING TO FRAME
IN INDOOR CLOTHING)

Height		Small Frame	Medium Frame	Large Frame
		Men		
Feet	*Inches*			
5	2	112–120	118–129	126–141
5	3	115–123	121–133	129–144
5	4	118–126	124–136	132–148
5	5	121–129	127–139	135–152
5	6	124–133	130–143	138–156
5	7	128–137	134–147	142–161
5	8	132–141	138–152	147–166
5	9	136–145	142–156	151–170
5	10	140–150	146–160	155–174
5	11	144–154	150–165	159–179
6	0	148–158	154–170	164–184
6	1	152–162	158–175	168–189
6	2	156–167	162–180	173–194
6	3	160–171	167–185	178–199
6	4	164–175	172–190	182–204

DESIRABLE WEIGHTS FOR WOMEN AGED 25 AND OVER (WEIGHT IN POUNDS ACCORDING TO FRAME IN INDOOR CLOTHING)

Height		Small Frame	Medium Frame	Large Frame
		*Women**		
Feet	*Inches*			
4	10	92– 98	96–107	104–119
4	11	94–101	98–110	106–122
5	0	96–104	101–113	109–125
5	1	99–107	104–116	112–128
5	2	102–110	107–119	115–131
5	3	105–113	110–122	118–134
5	4	108–116	113–126	121–138
5	5	111–119	116–130	125–142
5	6	114–123	120–135	129–146
5	7	118–127	124–139	133–150
5	8	122–131	128–143	137–154
5	9	126–135	132–147	141–158
5	10	130–140	136–151	145–163
5	11	134–144	140–155	149–168
6	0	138–148	144–159	153–173

* For girls between 18 and 25, subtract 1 pound for each year under 25.
(From Metropolitan Life Insurance Company)

Bibliography

Aftergood, L. and Alfin-Slater, R. B. "Women and Nutrition." *Contemporary Nutrition* 5 (1980).

Aftergood, L. "Dietary Fat—An Ongoing Controversy." *Nutrition and the M.D.* 8(1982):1.

Aker, S. and Lenssen, P. *A Guide to Good Nutrition During and After Chemotherapy and Radiation*, 2nd ed., 1979. Research Dietary Service, Division of Medical Oncology, Fred Hutchinson Cancer Research Center, 1124 Columbia Street, Seattle, WA 98104.

Albanese, A. A. Current Topics in Nutrition and Disease. Vol. 3. Nutrition for the Elderly. New York: Alan R. Liss, Inc., 1980.

" 'Alternative' Nutrition Therapies—Are They Safe?", *Environmental Nutrition Newsletter.* 5(1982):1.

"Anemia in the Elderly." *Nutrition and the M.D.* 6(1980):4.

"Animal Tests," *Carcinogen Information Program Bulletin*, no. 6, March 1979, Center for the Biology of Natural Systems, Washington University, St. Louis, Missouri.

"Antacid Osteomalacia," *Nutrition and the M.D.* 7(1981):5.

Appledorf, H. "How Good Are Fast Foods?" *Professional Nutritionist* 14(1982):1.

"Artificial and Alternate Sweeteners," *Nutrition and the M.D.* 7(1981):3.

Blum, M. and Elian, I. "The Vaginal Flora After Natural or Surgical Menopause." *Journal of American Geriatric Society*, 27(1979):395.

Bordia, A. "Effects of Garlic on Blood Lipid in Patients with Coronary Heart Disease." *American Journal Clinical Nutrition*, 34(1981):2100.

Breneman, J. C. "Food Allergy." *Contemporary Nutrition* 4(1979).

"Broiling and Benzo [a] Pyrene," *CIP Bulletin*, no. 2, August 1978.

"Caffeine." *Federal Register.* Part 6. 45(1980):69817. October 21, 1980.

"Caffeine: How to Consume Less." *Consumer Reports*, October 1981, p. 597.

"Caffeine: What It Does." *Consumer Reports*, October 1981, p. 595.

"The Calcium/Phosphorus Ratio." *Nutrition and the M.D.* 5(1979):4.

Cohen, S. "Pathogenesis of Coffee—Induced Gastrointestinal Symptoms." *New England Journal of Medicine.* 303(1980):122.

Cohn, S. D. "Vegetarian Nutrition: An Overview." *Health Care of Women* 1(1978):1.

"Composition of Foods, Dairy and Egg Products." *Agriculture Handbook no. 8–1*, USDA, Agricultural Research Service, U.S. Government Printing Office, Wash, D.C., 1976.

"Consultation: Treating Laetrile Toxicity." *Nursing 80*, September 1980, p. 90.

"Controlling Gaseousness." *The Health Letter*, 6(1975):1.

Coon, J. M. "Natural Food Toxicants—A Perspective." *Nutrition Reviews*, 32(1974):321.

Crapo, P. A. "Sugar and Sugar Alcohols." *Contemporary Nutrition*, 12(1981).

Darby, W. J. "Why Salt? How Much?" *Contemporary Nutrition.* 5(1980):1.

De Roin, N. R. "Coffee." *Restaurants and Institutions*, March 1981, p. 59.

Di Palma, J. R. and McMichael, R. "The Interaction of Vitamins with Cancer Chemotherapy." *CA-A Cancer Journal for Clinician* 29(1979):280.

Donegan, W. L. "The Association of Body Weight with Recurrent Cancer of the Breast." *Cancer* 41(1978):1590.

Dukes, J. E., et al. "Alcohol in Pharmaceutical Products." *American Family Physician*, September 1977, p. 97.

Dyerberg, J., et al. "Eiosapentaenoic Acid and Prevention of Thrombosis and Atherosclerosis" *Lancet*, 2(1978):117.

Eisele, J. W. and Reay, D. T. "Deaths Related to Coffee Enemas." *Journal of the American Medical Association.* 244(1980):1608.

Erhard, D. "The New Vegetarians, Part 2." *Nutrition Today*, 9(1974):20.

Everything Doesn't Cause Cancer, NIH Publication no. 79-2039, September 1979, National Cancer Institute.

Fenner, L. "Salt Shakes Up Some of Us." *FDA Consumer* 14(1980):2.

"Fluoride and Osteoporosis." *Nutrition and the M.D.* 5(1979):5.

"Food Colors: A Scientific Status Summary by IFT's Expert Panel on Food Safety and Nutrition." *Food Technology* 34(1980):77.

"Food Intolerances." *Nutrition and the M.D.* 6(1980):3.

Franklin, B. A. and Rubenfire, M. "Losing Weight Through Exercise." *JAMA* 244(1980):377.

Frazier, C. A. "Food Allergies." *Journal of Home Economics*, 69(1977):28.

Friedman, R. and Alfin-Slater, R. B. "Those Natural Toxins in Foods." *The Professional Nutritionist* 14(1982):5.

Georgakas, D. "How to Live Forever (Almost)." *CNI Weekly Report* 12(1982):4.

Gori, G. B. "The Cancer and Other Connections . . . If Any." *Nutrition Today* 16(1981):14.

Graedon, J. *The People's Pharmacy—2*, New York: Avon, 1980.

Gunby, P. "It's not fishy: fruit of the sea may foil cardiovascular disease," *Journal of the American Medical Association*, 247(1982):729.

"Hair Analysis—Use or Abuse?" *Nutrition and the M.D.* 7(1981):2.

Hall, R. L. "Safe as the Plate." *Nutrition Today*, 12(1977):6.

Hanington, Edda. "Diet and Migraine." *Journal of Human Nutrition* 34(1980):175.

"The Health Effects of Caffeine." American Council on Science and Health, 47 Maple Street, Summit, NJ 07901, March 1981.

"Health Practices Among Adults, United States, 1977." *Advance Data*, no. 64, November 4, 1980. Vital and Health Statistics of the National Center for Health Statistics, U.S. Department of Health and Human Services.

Hennekens, C. H. et al. "Daily Alcohol Consumption and Fatal Coronary Heart Disease," *American Journal of Epidemiology* 107(1978):196.

Herbert, V. and Selvey, N. "Amino-benzoic Acid: No Value in Human Nutrition." *JAMA* 243(1980):1092.

Hiermann, I. et al. "Effect of Diet and Smoking Intervention on the Incidence of Coronary Heart Disease." *Lancet*, December 12, 1981, p. 8259.

Hitt, C. "Risk Reduction: A Community Strategy." *Community Nutritionist*, January–February 1982, p. 12.

Holmes, T. H. and Rohe, R. N. "The Social Readjustment Rating Scale." *Journal of Psychosomatic Research* 11(1967):213.

Konishi, F. and Henderson, S. L. "Adult Requirements for Vitamin D. *Nutrition and the M.D.*, 7(1981):1.

Lantigua, R. A. et al. "Cardiac Arrhythmias Associated with a Liquid Protein Diet for the Treatment of Obesity." NEJM 303(1980): 735.

Larkin. T. J. "Drug Instruction: The Importance of Being Earnest." *FDA Consumer*, February 1976.

Leonard, R. E. "Workshop Examines Desirable Weights." *CNI Weekly Report* 12(1982):4.

Levine, Allen S. "The Relationship of Diet to Intestinal Gas." *Contemporary Nutrition* 4(1979):1.

Linksweiler, H. M. and Zemel, M. B. "Calcium to Phosphorus Ratios." *Contemporary Nutrition* 4(1979).

"MAOI Antidepressants vs. Tyramine-Containing Foods." *Nutrition and the M.D.* 5(1979):4.

Marcus, R. "Some Nutritional Aspects of Osteoporosis." *Nutrition and the M.D.* 5(1979):2.

McDonald, J. "Mixing Alcohol with Nutrition." *Professional Nutritionist* 3(1981):3.

Meister, K. A. "Mussels and Joints." *American Council on Science and Health Newsletter,* 2(1981):10.

"The Mistreatment of Arthritis." *Consumer Reports,* June 1979, p. 340.

Moertel, C. G. et al. "A Clinical Trail of Amygdalin (Laetrile) in the Treatment of Human Cancer." *NEJM* 306(1982):201.

Monro, J. et al. "Food Allergy in Migraine." *The Lancet,* July 5, 1980, p. 1.

"More than Alcohol alone . . . The Case for Wine." *Nutrition and the M.D.* 5(1979):4.

Natow, A. B. and Heslin, J. *Geriatric Nutrition,* Boston: CBI Publishing Co., 1980.

"The New Diet Pills." *Consumer Reports* 47(1982), p. 14.

"New Therapies, New Forms of an Old Vitamin." *Science News* 115(1979):181.

"Nutrition and the Fast Food Restaurant." *Nutrition and the M.D.* 5(1979):2.

"Nutrition and Menopause." *Environmental Nutrition News,* 2(1979):2.

"Older Problem Drinkers." *Alcohol Health and Research World,* Spring 1975, p. 12. National Institute on Alcohol Abuse and Alcoholism.

Oster, Kurt A. "Atherosclerosis, Conjectures, Data and Facts." *Nutrition Today* 16(1981):28.

Podolsky, S., El-Beheri, B. "The Principles of a Diabetic Diet." *Geriatrics* 35(1980):73.

Pops, M. A. "Peptic Ulcer Disease: Should You Prescribe a Diet?" *Nutrition and the M.D.,* 4(1978):1.

Position Paper on the Vegetarian Approach to Eating, *Journal of the American Dietetic Association* 77(1980):61.

"The Proper Treatment of Arthritis." *Consumer Report,* July 1979, p. 391.

Putnam, J. J. and Reidy, K. "Sodium: Why the Concern?" *National Food Review,* Summer 1981, p. 27.

Ravry, M. J., "Dietetic Food Diarrhea." *JAMA* 244(1980):270.

Robertson, L. et al. *Laurel's Kitchen.* New York: Bantam, 1978.

Rodman, M. J. "The Drug Interactions We All Overlook." *R.N.* April 1981, p. 61.

Rose, D. P. "The Pill and Nutrition: A Most Intricate Relationship." *Professional Nutritionist*, Summer 1977, p. 1.

Seaman, B. and G. *Women and the Crisis in the Sex Hormones.* New York: Rawson Associate Publishers, 1977.

"The Selling of H₂O." *Consumer Reports* 45(9) June 1980, p. 531.

Shekelle, R. B. et al. "Dietary Vitamin A and Risk of Cancer in the Western Electric Study." *Lancet*, November 28, 1981, p. 1185.

Simonson, M. "An Overview: Advances in Research and Treatment of Obesity." *Food and Nutrition News*, 53(1982):1.

Simpson, H. C. R. et al. "A High Carbohydrate Legumeous, Fibre Diet Improves All Aspects of Diabetic Control," *Lancet*, January 3, 1981, p. 8210.

Smith, C. H. (ed.) *Food Medications Interactions*, P. O. Box 26464, Tempe, AZ 85282, 1981.

Smith, E. B. "A Guide to Good Eating the Vegetarian Way." *Journal of Nutrition Education*, 7(1975):109.

The Sodium Content of Popular Prepared Food Items. Morton Salt Division of Morton Norwich Products, Inc., 110 North Wacker Drive, Chicago, IL 60606, no date.

Speer, F. *Food Allergy.* Littleton, Massachussetts: PSG Publishing. Co., 1978.

Speer, F. "Food Allergy: The 10 Common Offenders." *American Family Physician* 13(1976):106.

"Starch Blockers Classified as Drugs." *Community Nutrition Weekly Report*, XII (July 8, 1982):6.

Stephenson, P. E. "Physiologic and Psychotropic Effects of Caffeine on Man." *JADA*, 71(1977):240.

Stern, J. S. "Dining Out: How to Manage Calories." *Professional Nutritionist* 13(1981):11.

"Tastes of America." *Restaurants and Institutions* 89(1981):42.

Toxicants Occurring Naturally in Foods, 2nd. ed. Washington, D.C.: National Academy of Sciences, 1973.

"Vitamin B₁₅: Anatomy of a Health Fraud." American Council on Science and Health, September 1981.

"Vitamin Safety: A Factual Perspective." *Vitamin Issues* 11(1981):1.

"Which Comes First—Diet or Exercise?" *CNI Weekly Report* 9 (1979):4.

Zoumas, B. L. et al. "Theobromine and Caffeine Content of Chocolate Products." *Journal of Food Science* 45(1980):314.

Index

[The following codes are used throughout index: + = table; R = recipe; H = highlight box].